Assessing Aggression Thresholds in Dogs

Using the Assess-A-Pet Protocol to Better Understand Aggression

By Sue Sternberg

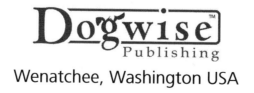

Wenatchee, Washington USA

Assessing Aggression Thresholds in Dogs

Using the Assess-A-Pet Protocol to Better Understand Aggression

Sue Sternberg

Dogwise Publishing

A Division of Direct Book Service, Inc.

403 South Mission Street, Wenatchee, Washington 98801

1-509-663-9115, 1-800-776-2665

www.dogwisepublishing.com / info@dogwisepublishing.com

© 2017 Sue Sternberg

Photos: Sue Sternberg

Graphic Design: Lindsay Peternell

Library of Congress Cataloging-in-Publication Data

Names: Sternberg, Sue, author.

Title: Assessing aggression thresholds in dogs : the revised Assess-a-Pet manual / by Sue Sternberg.

Description: Wenatchee, Washington : Dogwise Publishing, 2017. | Includes index.

Identifiers: LCCN 2016055137 | ISBN 9781617812033

Subjects: LCSH: Dogs--Behavior--Testing. | Aggressive behavior in animals--Testing. | Dogs--Psychology. | Dog adoption.

Classification: LCC SF433 .S74 2017 | DDC 636.7/089689142--dc23

LC record available at https://lccn.loc.gov/2016055137

ISBN: 978-1-6178120-3-3

Printed in the U.S.A.

DEDICATION

My parents, retired now, were both oncologists; my mother a pediatrician and my father a pathologist. Together, they worked over 80 years of combined service at Memorial Sloan Kettering Cancer Center in New York City.

They worked long hours. They didn't attend my recitals or watch me play basketball. I believe my first word was not "Mamma" or "Pappa" but rather, "Adriamycin." Talk at the family dinner table wasn't about school or homework, but rather disease and treatment and chemotherapy and radiation.

Growing up, I often longed for a more 'normal' upbringing, and dreamed of being raised in a more 'traditional' family (like, I always believed, Samantha and Darren Stevens offered from *Bewitched)*. It took me until I was an adult to realize what my parents gave me.

They valued honesty over everything. They scoffed at euphemisms.

My father founded and was chief editor for the *American Journal of Surgical Pathology,* and he hated euphemisms or haughty acronyms that could exclude someone from immediate clarity. While editing, he would always say, "It is not flatulence, it is farting."

My mother never spoke of a patient "passing away" but instead called it dying. She believed in speaking the truth, and using her actions and emotions to soften its impact or provide hope and support. She confronted a dismal 20% survival rate for children diagnosed with Non-Hodgkin's Lymphoma, and by changing the treatment protocols, improved the survival rate to 80%.

What I learned from my parents was to create a big and honest life—to work to make the world a better place. They inspired me have an impact, affect change, help people. To lay a foundation of truth, no matter how brutal, because it is only from that truth that the place exists in which to affect and create real change.

I dedicate this book to them, my amazing parents, who have always supported me and my path to make the shelter world a better place.

ACKNOWLEDGMENTS

It's truly a wonder I finished this book at all, what with my work and travel schedule, and how obsessed I have become with the sport of NACSW-Canine Nosework. On the other hand, it likely wouldn't have been written at all if it weren't for my involvement in the sport, and all the new friends it has made me. Dear friend Amy Herot (co-founder of the National Association of Canine Scent Work) came for a visit last year, and when I was lamenting about how I hadn't been able to get started revising my Assess-A-Pet program, how it was so long overdue, and how I was overwhelmed by the enormity of the project, she said quite simply, "Oh? I can help you get organized with that." And she pulled out her laptop, asked me questions, jotted down notes, asked me more questions, rearranged those notes, and then emailed me what she wrote. And it was like magic. Voila. All of a sudden the project was organized into discrete and doable chunks. Literally a few months later over three quarters of the manuscript was written, I had contacted Dogwise and this book was officially born. Thank you Amy. For everything.

A huge thank you to my friend and colleague Karen Owens, not just for the fun and friendship, but for always carrying the Assess-A-Pet torch, for being a science and data geek, videotaping everything, and never ceasing to care for your community as much as you do for the dogs. Special thank you to Karen and her colleagues Katy Johnson and Dana VanSickle at Charlotte-Mecklenburg Animal Care and Control for photos of assessments and dogs. And at the last minute.

Dr. Tim Lewis! Thank you for your contagious geekiness—for helping me think more like a scientist and hopefully behave more like one, too. And for going above and beyond the call of duty in scrutinizing and editing the manuscript. I'll pay you back in agates.

And thanks to the amazing team at Dogwise, who were somehow able to make sense of my sentences and thoughts—really 'get me'—and who were all so great to work with.

TABLE OF CONTENTS

Introduction...1

1. Assessing Aggression Thresholds: An Overview..3
2. Shelter Dogs and Adopters..6
3. Aggression Thresholds and Classifications..11
4. Aggression Threshold Testing Overview...13
5. The AAP Baseline Tests Step by Step...20
6. The Additional Tests—Step by Step..58
7. Assessing Aggression Thresholds in Owned or Fostered Dogs For Trainers and Behaviorists......................76
8. The Trinity: Dog-Human-Environment...95

Appendix 1: Research on Assessing Aggression Thresholds...99
Appendix 2: Glossary..101
Appendix 3: Observations from Video Reviews of Assessments...107
Appendix 4: Recommended Reading and Watching to Increase Your Knowledge of Dog Aggression,
   Body Language and Interactions...110
Appendix 5: Assessment Charts...111

About the Author..137
Index..139

INTRODUCTION

My original Assess-A-Pet manual, designed to help animal shelters determine which of their dogs were safe and appropriate for adoption, was published in 2006. Over time, the shelter dog population has changed considerably, and is far riskier today than ever before. In the drive to lower euthanasia rates and increase the live outcomes of more dogs, shelters are releasing into the community much more problematic—if not downright dangerous—dogs.

I began working on developing my own way to test the suitability of dogs for adoption soon after founding my own dog shelter in 1993. While I had done assessments on dogs for many years at shelters in the Northeast, I came to realize that I needed a more formal way to predict a dog's suitability as a pet. Each step, each response has been painstakingly created from real-life shelter dog experiences. The test was developed by deconstructing the most successful pet dogs and by studying and evaluating unsuccessful and returned dogs, as well as learning from dogs with a known behavior history. It is constantly being tweaked and revised as I hear back from shelter professionals who use the assessment, from people who have adopted, from people who can no longer keep their dog, from adopters I work with during behavior and training consultations, from my experiences fostering, as well as from my obsessive video studies of assessments.

How this book is organized
The book is divided into eight chapters:

1. Assessing aggression thresholds: an overview

2. Shelter Dogs and Adopters

3. Aggression Thresholds and Classifications

4. Aggression Threshold Testing Overview

5. The AAP Baseline Tests Step by Step

6. The Additional Tests—Step by Step

7. Assessing Aggression Thresholds in Owned or Fostered Dogs for Trainers and Behaviorists

8. The Trinity: Dog-Human-Environment

There are also five appendices at the back of the book including research on the methods presented in this book, a glossary, observations from video reviews of assessments and a recommended reading and viewing list. I have also included an extra set of all the Assessment Charts at the back of the book as well.

The newly revised Assess-A-Pet tests reflect not so much changes in the procedures of the original tests, but rather modifications designed to address the changing and evolving population of shelter dogs, and the changes in sheltering philosophies, goals and politics in this country. The protocols used to assess aggression thresholds I recommend had to evolve to address these changing safety concerns. I also wanted in this new book to address the needs of trainers, behavior professionals and rescue/foster personnel operating outside of the shelter environment, including those who offer in-home consultations. Many trainers, especially those hired to work with aggressive/reactive dogs, end up having to perform some type of assessment for their own safety when working with these dogs and to develop a training plan. You will find this information in the seventh chapter of the book.

CHAPTER 1

Assessing Aggression Thresholds: An Overview

The protocols I recommend in this book include a series of tests designed to determine a dog's aggression thresholds. These tests have for years been labeled under the name Assess-A-Pet (AAP) which have been updated and revised to better match today's shelter dogs and adopters. Temperament and behavior evaluations such as this help shelters determine which dogs are safe and appropriate for adoption or transfer, and which are too risky or downright dangerous to place back into the community. The temperament and behavior of each dog, rather than breed type, length of stay, or random, subjective decisions, should guide decisions about placement, transfer and euthanasia.

AAP measures aggression thresholds. The most successful pet dogs are ones with high aggression thresholds. Dogs with low aggression thresholds are not only at increased risk for aggression problems in the home, but just as often for more problematic behavior in the home, and more severe problem behaviors, even seemingly unrelated behaviors like separation anxiety, severe destructiveness, barking problems, reactivity and more.

AAP was specifically created by and for people evaluating and handling dogs in shelters, but can also be used by trainers and others who work with dogs in other environments. AAP assumes, and takes into account, the stressful and arousing nature of a shelter and kenneling. It does not penalize a dog for coming out of his kennel in an aroused state. Indeed, AAP assumes that shelter dogs have experienced a period of frustration, arousal, over-stimulation, deprivation and stress. The test is also designed to take into account the experiences particular to shelter dogs and to measure their responses. The responses you are looking for do not necessarily look like what you expect from an owned dog already settled in a home, nor are you looking always for overt aggressive responses.

The steps of AAP unfold in a specific order, each one building on the one before it. The test is deliberately laid out in this order not just to keep the tester safe, but to maximize each dog's potential for success.

The benefits of AAP:

- ❑ Allows shelter personnel, trainers and rescue personnel to interact more safely with dogs
- ❑ Allows you to better describe the dog's personality and temperament to prospective adopters
- ❑ Allows a trainer or staff person at a shelter to tailor training to each dog's strengths and weaknesses
- ❑ Helps the shelter determine where best to house/kennel each dog
- ❑ Allows shelter workers or trainers to counsel prospective adopters about potential behavior or training problems and ways to avert trouble

❑ Helps shelter workers or volunteers better understand and counsel people considering surrendering dogs, including those who may be dealing with difficult or even dangerous dogs

❑ Allows shelters to determine which dogs cannot safely be offered to the public

❑ Allows shelters to determine which dogs cannot safely be handled by volunteers

❑ Allows a shelter to provide whatever an adoptable dog needs to find a permanent, loving and appropriate home—whether that might be time, remedial care/treatment, behavior modification or transfer to a rescue group or another shelter with more adopters

❑ Allows a shelter to help keep their community safe, and to place out into society pet dogs that are safe, appropriate and successful—dogs that keep the rest of the humans, dogs and cats in the community safe from harm

❑ Can help a shelter make informed decisions that promote a more humane society

A brief history of assessments

When I first started working in shelters in 1981, decisions for adoption and euthanasia were made randomly—usually for length of stay, coat color (too many black and tan dogs) or breed type (back then it was Chows that held the worst reputation). In the early 1980s and before, dog trainers and behaviorists were not involved in the shelter world, nor were shelter people knowledgeable about training or behavior. These two main parts of the dog world were completely separate from each other. One had nothing to do with the other.

The public selects a dog for adoption by unknowingly reading a dog's body language, behavior and temperament. When asked why they chose a particular dog, the most common answer is, "Why, he chose me!" which translates into a mutual, sociable interaction. Potential adopters will wander down the kennel aisle, look hopefully into each kennel, bending over and sweet talking, while many dogs will be barking, lunging, jumping, hiding, pooping or whatever—and then there will be one sweet dog squeezed up against the front of the kennel, squinting, curled body, low tail wag, and interacting directly with the adopter. Sociability is what people mean when they say, "He chose me." People also return dogs for behavior and temperament reasons, even if what they write on the relinquishment form is, "Needs room to run," "Not enough time," "He got too big," etc. These are all generally behavioral issues.

Working in shelters and working as a dog trainer all at the same time helped me look at the shelter world through behavioral eyes. It seemed logical to me that decisions for placement and euthanasia should be based upon behavior and temperament.

I worked at the ASPCA (American Society for the Prevention of Cruelty to Animals) in the mid-1980s, when they were the agency responsible for animal care and control in New York City. Back then, the department called "Companion Animal Services" created a way to try to test temperament and make behavior decisions on the thousands of dogs coming in to the shelter, most of them strays with a 48-hour hold period before a euthanasia or adoption decision could be made. The sheer volume of incoming dogs put enormous time and space pressure on these dogs. Finding the best adoption candidates was so important; identifying the most dangerous dogs and limiting their exposure, handling and stress was equally important. Identifying the most risky dogs for euthanasia in order to have room for an incoming good pet dog was critical. I believe the ASPCA was one of the first organizations to perform any formal sort of assessment.

Back then, the professional dog training staff created and performed the assessments. Much of what was gleaned had to do with whether or not the dog should go to an "experienced dog owner," if it was considered a "dominant breed" of dog and therefore should go to an owner experienced with "dominant breeds," how "trainable" the dog seemed, and how the dog responded to the ambient noises and bustle of a big city. The biggest problem with what we did was that we handled and treated the dogs as professional dog trainers, and the dogs could not help but to respond to us as professionals—thereby eclipsing the way the dogs would communicate and behave for the average pet owner. Also, prior experience with a dog or a particular breed does not in any way guarantee an owner's ability to deal with a new dog. We were doing the best we could, but it had its limitations.

When I founded and opened my own shelter in 1993, I started by formally temperament testing only the "iffy" dogs, or ones whose behaviors my staff or I questioned. I assumed that with a "good eye" for dogs, and a thorough behavioral history upon intake from owner surrenders, I could pretty easily determine which dogs were probably okay. I also assumed that I could read a good dog, and that the ones that seemed the friendliest probably didn't need a formal assessment. I learned the hard way—by adopting out dogs that got returned by good people who were devastated by their experience, by adopting out a dog that seemed good but ended up biting someone. I learned the hard way (even harder for my adopters of dogs that didn't work out) that *every* dog should be assessed. First and foremost, every dog should be assessed because if the only dogs being assessed are the questionable ones, the test will appear skewed to staff and volunteers, and viewed as a way to "fail" or kill dogs. And secondly, if a professional sees something questionable in a dog, the likelihood that the dog will be suitable for the average family is already low.

Aggression, thankfully, while a huge problem *when* it occurs, is an *infrequent* event. You are unlikely to encounter that actual, infrequent aggressive event while the dog is in the shelter. To wait for overt aggression to predict overt aggression is, as I found out quite soon after working in shelters, a poor way to predict the future success of the dog in a home with real, non-professional dog owners.

CHAPTER 2

Shelter Dogs and Adopters

I used to divide adoptable dogs into three categories: Level One, Level Two and Level Three. Level One being the dogs with the highest aggression thresholds and therefore the easiest to live with successfully, Level Three being the most challenging dogs but still with high thresholds for aggression. There are corresponding levels of human adopters as well. Level One adopters are the least experienced and the least capable of managing and training a dog. Level Two are more capable and Level Three are skilled and experienced people, from hobby sports owners to professional trainers.

Level One makes up most of all adopters. They are generally inexperienced people with young children (age 7 and under) either already in the home, on the way into the home (the couple or individual is likely to have a new child come into the home within five years of adopting), or the people have young children in the environment, i.e., nieces and nephews, grandkids visiting, young children in the neighborhood riding bikes past, riding in the elevators, etc. People with young children have divided priorities and limited time to train and work with a dog. So they need a pretty bomb-proof dog that has tested out as having the least likely chances for serious problem behaviors, and has the highest aggression thresholds in all categories. This is the Level One dog. When available, they seem to originate from the rural South.

Over time, however, fewer and fewer Level One dogs are coming into shelters anywhere in this country, and in fact I believe the Level One dog to be very nearly extinct. So in this book, I have removed the Levels One, Two and Three classifications for dogs and converted the scoring from the least risky to the most risky. I have kept the Level One, Two and Three classifications for adopters.

I am guessing the near extinction of the Level One dog is due to more and more cooperation between shelters in the form of shelter transfers (from rural area southern shelters to more urban area shelters where there are better chances for adoption) and also more low-cost spay/neuter clinics and more aggressive spay/neuter campaigns. Also nobody is deliberately breeding for the Level One temperament pet dog. Nobody. Reputable purebred breeders sell their "pet quality" puppies (the ones that will live with real families with real children) under spay/neuter contracts, and keep intact for breeding stock dogs that typically are not proven pets (i.e., living successfully with families with young children). I am not saying reputable breeders aren't producing some great dogs, but very few are breeding first and foremost for this temperament—above and beyond the limitations of breed, physical looks and lack of conformation flaws. And those who are breeding for this are not breeding enough to influence the future of the pet dog. Plus, the temperament and behavior of the sweet, soft, deferential, highly sociable dog does not easily lend itself to the conformation show ring. It simply would not do to have the judge approach a dog and the dog to curl itself into a cashew shape, wag low and wide, squint his eyes, and maybe roll on his back. Or maybe the judges should be children…

Shelter dog populations

Shelters see the unwanted population in any community. In the 1970s, 1980s and in most areas of the United States also the 1990s, most shelters were dealing with dog *overpopulation*: too many dogs, not enough homes. Shelters were seeing many entire or almost entire litters of puppies (litters are the true marker of overpopulation). Each shelter, back then and just as much now, whether it formally performs temperament assessments or not, *places its best dogs up for adoption,* first and foremost. The public, knowing nothing formally about temperament, assessments or dog behavior, will themselves self-select the most friendly dog in any shelter dog population. But over the last few decades, the population of shelter dogs has changed, and we are seeing fewer and fewer behaviorally adoptable dogs.

As these numbers come down, the first portions of the dog population that shelters cease to see are the litters of puppies and the behaviorally adoptable dogs. There is huge demand for the supply of puppies, and so litters are no longer ending up in shelters. And, since adopting and rescuing has become more and more chic and "politically correct," it is not uncommon to hear owners of purebred dogs purchased from breeders admitting that they feel embarrassed/ashamed, reluctant to admit to having purchased rather than rescued/saved a dog. The result is that in most regions of the country there are more adopters for safe pet dogs than there are safe pet dogs in shelters.

Shelters place up for adoption their most adoptable dogs—with or without a formal assessment. Whether it is by "eye-balling" the dogs' behaviors, or by kennel behavior or veterinary information during intake, shelters are still trying to place the best dogs in the population. But the best dog today is a very different dog from the best dog from a decade or two decades ago. The most behaviorally adoptable dog in the shelter today is a dog who, ten years ago, would, in all likelihood, have been considered at best a problematic candidate for adoption, not an easy, sweet, soft pet dog. Many dogs today that shelter professionals label as a gray area or more problematic dog, are dogs that ten years ago may have been euthanized for being too difficult, risky or dangerous to adopt out, especially in shelters with space and time limitations. But today, these dogs are ending up on the adoption floor and getting adopted out, or being transferred out to rescue groups. Or, in the current and potent "no-kill" climate, these problematic and risky dogs are living their lives out in shelters all over the country and the world.

Over time, shelters are unknowingly and unwittingly lowering the bar on what temperament of dog will make the safest and most successful pet dog. Because we are simply no longer seeing sociable pet dogs, we are identifying candidates for adoption by defining sociability and pet-suitability based on the least aggressive dogs in the facility. In many high-crime-area shelters, it has been so long since the shelter has encountered a sociable dog that people no longer know what sociability looks like, or worse, that it even ever existed.

Shelter live release rate trends

What does the term "live release rate" mean? The term comes from the Asilomar Accords, which are standards of practice developed and written in 2004 by a gathering of 18 local, regional and national animal welfare leaders. Its aim was to standardize shelters' record keeping and to help promote statistical recording for better tracking of shelter populations, with the ultimate aim of helping to end the euthanasia of healthy and treatable animals. A live release is any animal that exits the shelter alive—whether via adoption, being returned to an owner, transferred out to a rescue group or relocated to another shelter. A shelter's annual live release rate is calculated by dividing the total live outcomes (adoptions, outgoing transfers, return to owners) by the total outcomes (total live outcome plus euthanasias excluding owner-requested euthanasias).

Upon intake, animals are classified as healthy, treatable or rehabilitatable, and these refer to the animal's physical as well as behavioral health. A dog who is considered dangerous to humans or other animals in the community is not supposed to be considered healthy, treatable or rehabilitatable. But therein lies the subjectivity.

The trend currently is for shelters to increase their live release rates. This, of course, sounds like a "good" goal. However, if we understand what is happening to the overall temperaments of current populations of shelter dogs, and what is happening to the percentages of behaviorally adoptable dogs, this may appear instead to be a risky trend.

I have observed that a shelter's population of dogs has always been influenced by local crime rates. Shelters in higher crime areas have historically always had more aggressive dogs. Shelters in urban environments have always had a higher ratio of aggressive dogs to behaviorally adoptable ones than in more rural area shelters. The percentages of guarding and fighting breed types in shelters all over the country, rural and urban, seem to have increased. It is to the point where many shelters see almost exclusively guarding and fighting mixes (with more and more Chihuahua type dogs showing up). The dogs that shelter professionals are making decisions on are, for the most part, so much more aggressive, more muscular, larger and more risky than ever before. AAP is constantly being revised to reflect that risk whenever there are parts of the test I no longer consider safe to execute. My goal originally was to test dogs for placement as safe and successful pet dogs. Since there are so few behaviorally appropriate pet dogs in shelters today, and shelter professionals always are trying to select their "best" dogs for placement, over time, the criteria for what makes a "best" dog, or what makes for a safe pet, has morphed and adjusted itself to fit the changing population, instead of the changing population affecting the live release rate.

It is my experience that shelters are routinely placing dogs that pose high risk for aggression toward humans and other animals. Every shelter strives to increase its live release rate. All too often, behavior staff is pressured to try to classify more dogs as treatable or rehabilitatable, or approve the dog for transfer out to a rescue group or another shelter instead of euthanasia, to avoid negatively affecting the shelter's live release rate.

If the behavior and temperament of a shelter's dog population have been getting more risky and dangerous and there is managerial pressure to increase the shelter's live release rate, how can this be achieved? Most shelters I have visited solve this dilemma by transferring out to rescue for placement or placing high-risk dogs into the community. And very little follow-up is conducted. The rare follow-up that is conducted often only records "returns" in the first 30 days of adoption. After one month, recordings of dogs returned are classified as "owner-surrenders." I find this irresponsible.

The behavior and temperament of the dogs must trump the need for high or increasingly higher live release rates. If ten dogs in a shelter are assessed on a particular day, and all ten test out as dangerous, it does not make the slightly less dangerous dogs of the lot more adoptable because the percentage or proportion of dogs has to remain at a certain rate. Public safety is public safety. We may not like what the results of a temperament test show us, but adjusting the outcomes to improve a shelter's statistics, or in the name of "no-kill," or worse, to avoid the truth of the sheer number of difficult and dangerous dogs in our shelters is irresponsible, immoral and unconscionable.

The biggest problem is that there are far fewer behaviorally adoptable dogs in shelters today, and far more aggressive ones than anyone—public or within the shelter and rescue industry—is prepared to deal with.

Regional differences in shelter dog populations

We are quite successfully spaying and neutering all the best dogs, and our shelters are filling with the last population of dogs whose owners resist spaying and neutering: the working and sporting dogs in any community. In the rural areas, the working dog is a ranch-work and farm-work, livestock herding or guarding dog, etc. Sporting dogs are hunting (either with gun dogs, pointers, setters, spaniels, retrievers) or hunting with scent or sight hounds. Dogs of these breed types and profiles generally are bred to work with and around humans, and they exhibit a fairly low level of aggression to humans and other dogs. The rural sporting and working dogs tend to have high aggression thresholds, and a natural connection/affinity toward humans and other dogs.

The southern portion of the United States has bigger populations of dogs overall. Since they have warmer weather, more dogs are living or staying outdoors year-round, and thus there are two potential breeding cycles a year. In the northern rural areas, dogs can't survive as well outdoors in the cold, and hence they have one breeding season, and fewer litters per year.

In urban areas, and areas with high crime, the sport is dog fighting, and the work is guarding. So, more urban or higher crime area shelters are filled with guarding and fighting type bull-breed dogs: larger, more muscular and athletic dogs with lower thresholds for aggression, both to humans and to other dogs.

With so many guarding and fighting breed types, shelter dog populations today have much more potential for serious aggression, and are much more capable of doing harm. These dogs, *if* they are going to be aggressive in the community, are likely to have a more severe event as compared to populations of dogs 20 years ago. And today, this is the pool of dogs that shelter staff and volunteers are choosing from when trying to identify the most adoptable dogs in the shelter.

Why does it seem that the sweetest, softest, most biddable and sociable dogs come from the rural southern parts of the country? It is a phenomenon not noticed just by me. Shelter and training professionals who work with lots of rural southern dogs as well as northern dogs can often tell the difference as well. There is a visual, behaviorally palpable and observable quality to many of these dogs. I am sure this is a measurable quality, but I just don't know what to measure. Someone should study it.

I have a hypothesis about why this occurs. Or maybe less of a hypothesis and more of a question. What if the formula for breeding a sweet, soft, sociable dog is not merely to use only a sweet, soft, sociable sire and dam, but also to keep the gestating dam in a quiet, tranquil environment, maybe even outdoors, with the sounds of nature (crickets, frogs, birds) instead of traffic, neighbors fighting, noises and lots of people? What if the formula for producing sweet, soft, sociable dogs is not to socialize and provide early neural stimulation and expose the puppies to noise and surface stressors but rather the elements of peace and quiet and safety that a warm, rural environment provides?

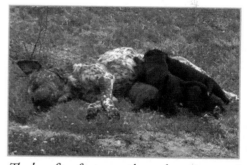

The benefits of a tranquil, rural environment?

There are dogs that shelter professionals encounter that the rest of the dog world don't even know exist: sweet, soft, sociable dogs so easy to raise and be with that trainers never see them because the owners report that the dogs don't seem to need training—that they already "listened" to them, and behaved in such a way naturally that official training seemed redundant. There are sweet, soft, sociable dogs that don't get early socialization (often spend their formative months in a backyard) yet come out as late as five, six or seven months and end up coping just fine with noises and novel stressors.

Maybe instead of emphasizing socialization and early training we should first emphasize the breeding of dogs that need less socialization and less rigorous training (although I believe all dogs benefit from both, for life) to be successful with the average person. After all, we are responsible for dogs, we are not held captive by the way things are.

Understanding the adopters

People who work or volunteer in shelters are often quite different from the average adopter. What they are able to live with, manage and tolerate can be quite different from what the average person or family wants or is able to manage and live with.

Level One adopters

The majority of adopters are basically inexperienced; they may or may not have had a dog before, but they are not professional trainers nor proficient in reading behaviors and body language. These adopters may take a training class or two, but they do not have the time or interest to become skilled dog trainers and handlers. They will not have the time, skill or experience to manage a seriously problematic dog. These adopters react and respond to their dog's behavior well into a behavioral sequence or very often at the end of a behavioral sequence. For example, the dog on the leash of the average adopter sees another dog on leash approaching at a distance; the dog orients toward the other dog, puts his ears forward, tenses up, steps forward, tightens the leash, begins growling, lunging and barking at the other dog, working himself up into a frenzy—which is often when the average adopter intervenes in the problem behavior and pulls his dog away. The professional dog owner sees the approaching dog appear, captures his own dog's attention, moves briskly away or skirts around the other dog, and sees no barking/growling/lunging. Experienced dog trainers thwart and manage behavioral sequences and ensure a good outcome; inexperienced owners react only after undesirable behavior has already occurred.

Level One adopters need dogs with the highest aggression thresholds in *all* categories of aggression. Single people or couples with even the potential for young children in the environment need dogs without any red-flag or problematic behavior, and need dogs with big, high aggression thresholds.

Level Two adopters

Level Two adopters are not professional dog trainers. Nor do they fall into the category of Level One owners. Level Two adopters fall somewhere in between. They may be people who have never owned a dog before but who have a natural leadership and calm countenance. The Level Two adopter tends to read behaviors extremely well, in people and in dogs, and has internally established rules and pre-organized guidelines for how a dog should behave, which in turn creates a more stable and clear environment.

Level Two adopters can often handle a slightly more assertive, clever, anxious, pushy or challenging dog. They may not necessarily like pushier or anxious dogs, but they may be more capable of handling them successfully. Level Two adopters should, in general, have no children under age 7, or if they do, the one young child should be very mature and gentle.

Level Three adopters

Level Three adopters can be professional dog trainers, shelter workers or handlers, vet techs, animal control officers or regular pet owners who are hobby dog sports enthusiasts—people for whom dogs are the central theme in their lives. They generally have excellent timing and the ability and desire to intervene early in a behavioral sequence, often unconsciously cutting off behaviors before they occur. The Level Three owner holding the leash of the dog described earlier would hear the dog tags of the approaching dog at the same time as her dog hears it, feel her dog become alert, and would then interrupt the sequence, either consciously by calling the dog or unconsciously by petting the dog or tugging the leash just enough to break the dog's attention off the other dog.

CHAPTER 3

Aggression Thresholds and Classifications

Aggression is the most challenging and difficult behavior to modify in dogs. The liability, both emotional and financial, of living with an aggressive dog is profound. At my shelter, I have learned that people rarely return a dog for frivolous or easy-to-solve behavior problems, such as house-training or mild, normal adolescent destructive chewing. It does happen, but dogs with low aggression thresholds have more non-aggressive behavior problems—and those behavior problems are more severe—as well as having aggression problems, and this is a common reason for return or surrender. And aggression is the one problem that people coming to adopt a dog do not want to work with. I divide aggressive behaviors into four classifications for the purpose of testing aggression thresholds below.

1. Handling and frustration aggression

Aggression can arise in a variety of situations in the home. Aggression due to handling or frustration—directed toward familiar people or family members when the dog is made to do something he doesn't want to do, or prevented from doing what he does want to do—is one of the most common forms of aggression in the pet dog and the most difficult threshold to predict in shelter dogs without doing a formal and valid temperament test.

Handling and frustration aggression reveals itself in many common situations: the dog is on the couch and the owner tries to push him off or move him so the owner can sit down; the dog is trying to go out the front door, or has his head in the trash, and the owner takes him by the collar to prevent him from doing these things; it is raining outside and the owner goes to wipe down the dog's feet with a towel; the owner attempts to put ointment in the dog's ears, etc. These are all common situations that occur and can result—for the dog with low thresholds for handling and frustration—in growling, snapping or biting, even hospitalizing, and, yes, even killing the owner.

In one case, nail clippers were found next to the dead owner of a Doberman recently adopted from one shelter, suggesting an extreme form of this type of aggression.

Dogs with low thresholds for handling and frustration aggression can be particularly dangerous with children who are usually unable to alter or inhibit their own behavior after just a mild warning from the dog. Most warnings are missed by inexperienced people, and especially by children.

I believe that the higher the sociability score (covered in detail starting on page 33), the higher the thresholds are for handling/frustration type aggression; the lower the sociability score, the lower the aggression thresholds. Sociability seems to act as a buffer.

2. Resource guarding

Resource guarding is another common form of aggression. Sometimes, the dog with handling and frustration aggression also competes for and guards valued resources in the home. It could be a chewable bone/toy, a food bowl, a chicken bone snatched from the sidewalk, the open dishwasher loaded with greasy, food-encrusted plates, or a pork-roast cooling on the kitchen counter. A valued resource could be something we consider inedible or inconsequential, but to the dog, it is highly desired or important—for instance the TV remote control, a shoe, an eyeglass case, the car, or the dog's crate. A highly valued resource could be the owner, and the dog stands between the owner and any other approaching human.

A dog's guarding resources from other dogs or the family cat does not necessarily predict that he will guard resources from humans. However, dogs that guard resources from humans almost always guard from other dogs or animals as well. A dog that guards resources from other dogs/animals usually needs to be placed more carefully into a home that already has a dog, but I have seen no direct correlation between dogs that guard against other dogs and dogs that will guard against children or adult humans.

3. Aggression toward strangers

Sometimes fear-based, sometimes not, sometimes a further manifestation of resource guarding, sometimes not, aggression directed toward non-family members poses the greatest financial liability for the pet owner, not to mention it makes for a highly stressful lifestyle trying to anticipate the behavior of every guest, visitor or stranger. From a dog training and behavioral standpoint, aggression toward strangers is a particularly hard issue to manage successfully, since it requires controlling and managing the behavior of other people, including strangers whom you've not met yet, and don't know what they're going to do until they do it.

4. Dog-dog aggression

Dog-dog aggression, when serious enough and exhibited by a dog physically capable of doing harm, poses a threat to society and the community. There really is no environment where the dangerous dog will not encounter someone else's dog. Even a visit to the veterinarian requires waking through the lobby or reception area, which can be filled with waiting dogs.

Dogs with serious aggression toward other dogs are, at best, destined to live very restricted lifestyles—usually unable to go for walks or hikes in public places, unable to go off leash in parks or on trails, unable to attend group dog training classes, etc. Also, practically every dog will get loose in his lifetime, and since such a dog may cause serious injury or death to another dog, it is irresponsible and unconscionable to place a seriously dog-aggressive dog in the community. These consequences must be considered when evaluating dogs for adoption.

CHAPTER 4

Aggression Threshold Testing Overview

The AAP test is gentle and non-confrontational. It does not threaten the dog in any way or cause pain. For the most part, it consists of observation and procedures that mimic what might happen to an average dog in average and common situations. The test helps reveal a lot about the dog's personality, needs and adoptability. Properly done, it will provide a shelter professional information about a dog's aggression thresholds and the risks posed by the dog in a variety of situations.

Having concrete, observable signs allows the tester to validate test results to others. It takes opinion out of decision-making at the shelter. It separates the person who is testing the dog from the evaluation and outcome, and allows decisions to be based on consistent test methodology and data, not on emotion. Remember, there is no one to blame for an unadoptable dog.

Before getting into the details, a quick important note: Testing should never be done alone, for the safety of the tester and also because more than one person is needed to test and observe the dog. The ideal is to have one helper to observe and record all of the dog's responses, or to have all the assessments video recorded for future reference.

Gathering what you need
Here is a list of equipment and supplies for using AAP in shelters:

A 6-foot leather or cloth-rope noose lead. In working with unknown dogs, the safety benefits of a leather or cotton noose lead, as opposed to the thin, 3-foot nylon slip leads so often found in shelters, are unparalleled. Leather or cotton is more comfortable on your hands, offers a better grip, and if an emergency muzzle is necessary, leather and cotton are easier to manipulate and stay more securely on the dog. I recommend the width be a minimum of 5/8 inches, and the length ideally 6 feet. The width is more comfortable on a dog's throat and causes less gagging and choking, and is less likely to be considered a correction by a dog that jerks suddenly. The 6-foot length affords the handler a variety of distances in which to handle and interact with the dog. A noose lead is easy to get on a dog. It requires a minimum of fuss and confrontation—a dog can walk into a noose on his own, and does not need a handler to reach down, lean over and deal with the dog's neck—and it allows the handler to maintain a neutral, gentle, steady tension on the line. The combination of leather or cotton, a 6-foot length, and the noose allows the handler to manage and maneuver the dog without informing the dog of his or her own expertise as a trainer or handler, and only influences the behavior of the dog minimally.

A chair to be used in the Sociability and Stranger tests.

A blanket or large towel used to provide a resting area for the dog during the Resource Guarding tests.

Assess-A-Hand. The Assess-A-Hand (see photos on page 41) was invented decades ago for shelter workers needing a safe way to test dogs for resource guarding without risking their own hands. Prior to the invention of the AAH, shelter workers typically used their feet to kick around the food bowl, or a broomstick to poke at the bowl while the dog ate. These options are not only an inaccurate assessment of the dog's responses, but unfair, as a dog might feel especially threatened by a gesture that looks like a kick, as well as have prior traumatic experiences with broomsticks, or at least be afraid of them.

Large dog food bowl filled to the brim with a mixture of dry kibble and canned food, mixed thoroughly so a dog cannot pick out choice morsels.

Pig's ear, Greenie or beef-basted bone, something the dog will consider valuable and start chewing when you hand it to him, and something that is long-lasting.

Rope or cloth toy, preferably at least a foot in length, which allows the dog to have his mouth on the toy but still leaves room for the tester to hold the toy.

Life-sized infant baby doll, preferably one that makes life-like baby noises.

Life-sized toddler sized doll, preferably one with a realistic face and a body that can be manipulated to look like a real child approaching.

Life-sized, realistic stuffed dog.

A realistic, fake cat, preferably one that mechanically moves and can make realistic cat like noises.

Who should do the testing

Testing should be done by skilled and experienced professional dog handlers and, again, should never be done alone, both for safety and because it takes more than one person to test and observe the dog. Two or three testers are ideal.

Testers familiar with or already emotionally attached to the dog being tested usually cannot be objective and, therefore, should not test that dog. In addition, testers who have already revealed their own level of competence and professional skill in handling a particular dog cannot effectively test, as the dog will likely then only respond as it would to a professional, not the average inexperienced pet owner.

The most common reason temperament tests can be invalid in predicting behavior in the home is because the tester handles the dog like a professional and skilled dog handler. Most adopters are not as skilled and confident when handling or living with dogs, which is why it is vital that testers must hide who they really are when testing the dogs. Assess-A-Pet attempts to keep the skill level of the tester anonymous so true responses can be obtained from the dog.

When to test

AAP should be done after the dog has had at least three days, ideally four, to settle into the shelter environment. Studies have shown that stress hormone levels drop after three days in a kennel environment. While AAP does not necessarily penalize a dog for being stressed, there are two important reasons to wait the minimum period:

1. Fearful and sensitive dogs may be overly traumatized by their experience arriving at the shelter; they may show behaviors that could penalize them during testing (hiding, lethargy, disconnected, owner-searching, etc.). Waiting four days can help these dogs acclimate.

2. Aggressive and dangerous dogs also need time to settle in and get more comfortable, because in the first few days they might appear friendly and perhaps benign, not coming anywhere near an aggression threshold. After settling into the territory and getting more comfortable, however, they show a more accurate picture of their temperament. Low threshold resource guarders need time to settle in and count the environment and things in it as their own.

Where to test

Testing should be done indoors and in a quiet environment. The testing room should be as comfortable and quiet as possible, with the fewest possible distractions and interruptions. Testing should be done away from other dogs and out of the kennels. If for some reason a shelter has no discrete indoor location, a quiet outdoor location (away from other dogs/distractors) is better than not testing at all. Most shelters have a bathroom, and this can be used as a testing room if there is no other indoor space.

Which dogs should be tested

Ideally, no dog should be put up for adoption without first being tested. If a shelter has just started to try to implement a temperament-testing program even for just a few dogs, it is most important to test the dogs that seem the most friendly and adoptable, as well as all the puppies. All puppies should be tested because they are most likely to be selected by the public for adoption, and are also most likely to be adopted by families with young children, so safety and compatibility of dog and family is of the utmost concern.

The priority is to locate the most adoptable dogs, to place them up for adoption and to keep them from being euthanized. If they do not get adopted quickly, these are dogs for whom rescue or transfer may be a priority.

The most common mistake shelters make is to use temperament testing only for the "iffy'" or questionable dogs. This is unwise for two reasons: One, it will skew the testing so that it will fail most dogs. Two, it uses the shelter's precious time and resources to test dogs already found to be questionable by professionals, while the temperament of dogs going out into our communities remains unknown.

If a shelter perceives a lack of sufficient time to devote to assessments, their priority should be to assess the most seemingly adoptable dogs: the puppies, the friendliest-*seeming*, and any dog the public is most likely to want to adopt. A shelter needs to know the behavior and temperament of the dogs that are most likely to go out into the community. Sheltering is not just about producing impressive "numbers" and good adoption "statistics." Sheltering is not just about being an adoption "boutique," or having low euthanasia numbers, or high adoption or transfer numbers. Dogs are not numbers. The community at large takes precedence over "numbers." Never has this been more important than today, when many of the dogs we are seeing are larger, more muscular, often neither bred nor raised as family pets, and therefore capable of doing great harm. Community safety is not just a goal for animal services or government/municipal facilities. Community safety is a responsibility and a goal that belongs to all of us.

At what age can a dog be tested?

If the dog is old enough to be adopted, the dog should be tested. I have many reports and anecdotal evidence from shelters that do not routinely test their puppies, that the bulk of their returned adoptions are 7- to 8-month-old dogs that were adopted out as unevaluated young puppies. I have found better accuracy at 8 weeks than at 7 weeks, so I recommend waiting to test and adopt out at 8 weeks. The only differences in using Assess-A-Pet on puppies as opposed to adult dogs is that many puppies are not leash trained and may be tested off leash (in a small area using an ex-pen to limit space around the tester similar to a leash). Puppies 4 months and younger should skip the Stranger Test, and can be tested with the tester kneeling or squatting instead of standing for the four Sociability tests.

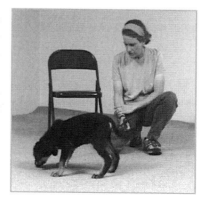

Test outline

As I have mentioned, the AAP test is a carefully laid out sequence, with each part building on the last. If the dog fails a step, the test is stopped. The details of each step are included in the next chapter.

There are four parts of the base test:

1. Cage Presentation

2. Sociability

3. Resource Guarding

4. Dog-Dog Aggression

In an ideal world, every shelter would fully assess every dog (safety issues allowing) with the base and all the additional tests. The base test gives the most crucial information. Additional tests may be called for under various circumstances. If a shelter has the time and resources, adding the Teeth Exam and the Stranger test to the base tests is preferred. See Chapter 5 for details on the additional tests.

Cage Presentation

The test starts, quite naturally, with **Cage Presentation:** observing the dog in his kennel. Any cage and barrier aggression is identified at this point in the test. The Cage Presentation test is used to screen for dogs likely too risky to even take out of the kennel for testing. While observing dogs in their kennels/cages may allow you to identify dogs with aggression thresholds too *low* to be suitable pets, you cannot accurately identify dogs with aggression thresholds high enough to be deemed suitable pets. Hence, it is necessary to take those dogs out of their kennels/cages for continued testing.

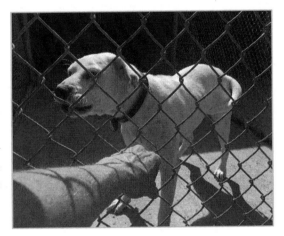

Sociability

The next four steps make up the **Sociability** section of the test and are extremely important signposts for evaluating the dog's responses later on in the test. The four sociability sub-tests are:

1. **Stand and ignore for 60 seconds**

2. **Three back strokes**

3. **Sit in a chair**

4. **20 seconds of attention**

A dog's Sociability score has direct influence on the dog's Resource Guarding scores. Dogs that score an 8 or higher in sociability and freeze or freeze/growl during either of the last two tests of the Resource Guarding tests are, in my experience, less risky than dogs that score 7 and under in Sociability and have the same responses during Resource Guarding tests.

Why test for sociability?

Sociability is defined as a dog's tendency to seek a friendly, congenial and affectionate interaction with humans. It does not refer to "socialization," which is the period of exposure, training and habituation to novel stimuli (humans, noises, environment) during critical periods of puppy development, but rather sociability is the aspect of a dog's temperament in which he seeks affable, affectionate and deferential relationships with humans.

Lack of sociability is one of the best indicators of future aggression. In fact, studies that have evaluated the usefulness of assessing aggression threshold tests show a significant correlation between lack of sociability and problem and aggressive behaviors.

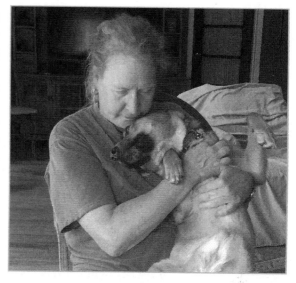

Sociability and true friendliness seem to act as buffers against aggression. Most aggression toward humans appears in the form of aggression around handling, being made to do something the dog does not want to do, or when preventing the dog from doing what he does want to do. If a dog seeks out, enjoys and finds pleasurable rewarding human touch, praise, affection, companionship (not just treats and toys), when the time comes to change pleasure petting into unpleasant handling—pulling out a tick or grooming out a tangle, or anything the dog deems unpleasant or unwanted—the dog is less likely to reach an aggression threshold. The sociable dog that seems to love to be touched and enjoys being held will seek out and relax during hugs from humans, instead of biting people who hug them.

For the dog that merely tolerates petting, or isn't internally rewarded by human praise, touch or affection, anything the dog finds unpleasant or unwanted can cause the him to reach his aggression threshold quickly.

If there were one part of aggression threshold assessments more important than any other, it would be the four Sociability tests. These are usually the least dramatic responses, rarely eliciting any flashy, overt aggressive displays, and yet the lack of sociability in a dog is often the most significant indicator of the dog's potential for lack of success in a home.

Sociability is not about how shy or outgoing a dog is. It is a temperament trait that also helps measure aggression thresholds. You live with temperament, you train the dog. The goal is never to *train* the dog to be more sociable. Sociability is a trait that is part of temperament and refers to a dog's basic willingness to socialize with and defer to humans, and has nothing to do with "socialization." Training a dog to approach the owner more often or approach the owner non-frontally, or trying to condition the dog to accept petting, is irrelevant. The goal in any training plan—*after having determined that the situation is indeed workable* and it is safe to design and begin implementing a training plan—is to give the dog more vocabulary for better communication, to increase the access to joy and fun that the owner(s) can offer the dog. This might include partnered outdoor recreation such as hiking or biking, dog sports that allow for instincts to be expressed like nosework, agility training, etc., and playing with the dog, thereby gaining respect from the dog by increasing the number of ways the dog *needs* the owner(s) for his own survival as well as fun. Dogs will develop more of a bond with owners they need, desire to be with, respect and by whom they are not threatened.

Resource Guarding

The third section of the test is designed to assess **aggression thresholds for resource guarding.** While the *tests* themselves look specifically at responses to a cloth toy, a chewable toy and a food bowl, the *responses* predict any kind of guarding aggression problems, from territorial to owner guarding.

The procedures for the AAP Resource Guarding tests are laid out in a very particular order, with only the very last step having anything to do with pushing the dog away from his resource. The steps (detailed in Chapter 5) are designed to communicate to the dog the desire for the tester to compete for the resource. The tester begins by taking a large and deliberate step forward toward the dog—one foot steps forward and the other foot steps to meet and align with the first. This clearly communicates to the dog that the tester is not just randomly or casually moving, but rather deliberately approaching the resource and observing the dog's competitiveness or deference.

The next steps mimic the way most pet owners interact with a dog in a home in which the dog has some access to resources. The dog has some resource he considers highly valuable, of which the owner is unaware. The dog has or is guarding said resource, the owner comes over to love on/interact innocently with the dog and then the dog responds. So the next tests involve the tester petting, stroking and praising the dog first on the back and then on the dog's head, closer to the resource.

The hesitant communication issue

The next steps are the most crucial to—and the very crux of— evaluating a dog's responses to high-value resources. It involves what I call **hesitant communication** on the part of the tester. It is the communication of hesitation that triggers the conflicted resource guarder. The hesitant communication during the approach to a resource is exactly how a child approaches a dog. The hesitant communication is exactly how the novice dog owner approaches a dog with a valued resource. The hesitant communication is exactly how the new dog owner approaches his new dog when he doesn't yet know or completely trust him. And it is exactly how the dog with low thresholds will be triggered into an aggressive state.

This is why a dog can show aggression during his resource guarding tests, and then a rescue group pulls the dog from the shelter and places him into a foster home, but the foster person scorns the assessments and reports back, "Why, I can reach right in there and take anything away from the dog!"

Highly experienced people, confident and smooth around dogs will reach toward a dog engaged with a valued resource with one fluid motion, and a deep, internal attitude of "don't you dare show me any problems here, buddy...." Aggressive events occur when the outcome of a particular situation is up for grabs or uncertain. When the dog believes *without a doubt* he can keep his valued resource, he will not waste calories in an aggressive display. When a dog believes he would surely lose his valued resource, he will not risk calories or harm in trying to defend it. When the outcome is uncertain? The dog is most likely to risk aggression. On either side of the bell curve of uncertainty is the neutral event. In the midst of controversy—where the possibility exists of a win or a loss—is where the aggression will ignite.

That is why the steps for the Resource Guarding tests are so crucial to assessing the dog's thresholds. Also, the earlier in the sequence the dog hits his aggression threshold, I believe the more risky the dog. Dogs that hit a threshold during the last step (while pushing the dog's muzzle away) I believe are less risky than dogs that freeze during the approach or during stroking.

Dog-Dog Aggression

The fourth section of the AAP test is **Dog-Dog Aggression.** Some shelters are currently starting with the Dog-Dog tests since they see such a high percentage of serious dog-dog aggression, and they use this test as a screen-out. This is acceptable.

If a dog shows risky behaviors in one portion, it is risky, if not dangerous, for the tester to continue testing. The test is laid out in an order best designed for tester safety. The base tests are fairly low risk for testers and helpers. The additional tests pose an increased risk for the tester and helper, particularly if testers pursue each test despite seeing risky and highly risky responses.

How long does the Assess-A-Pet test take?

The time it takes to assess a dog varies greatly from shelter to shelter, as included in that time is the distance from the kennels to the testing room. The dog-dog portion of the test tends to take the longest, as it involves two people, and may need to be repeated with more than just one dog, and/or the fake, stuffed dog. In regions of the country where shelters see a high volume of dog-aggressive dogs, evaluators start with the dog-dog test and use it as a rule-out in the interest of time, as they don't place dangerously dog-aggressive dogs into their communities. The current AAP baseline test takes an average of ten minutes per dog to complete. Some shelters halt testing if a dog shows high-risk behaviors; some shelters continue testing each dog fully. The baseline test plus all the additional tests takes an average of 15 to 20 minutes per dog.

The priority for any shelter is to identify all the adoptable dogs, test them and get them on the adoption floor. Shelters overwhelmed with incoming dogs should prioritize the test for their most "friendly" and "highly-adoptable" seeming dogs—as these are the ones the public will usually select first. These are the dogs most likely to go out into the community, and they should be known quantities. Also, identifying the most adoptable dogs first allows the shelter to contact rescue groups or other shelters willing and able to transfer in dogs, as well as identifying those dogs with treatable physical health issues that could (and should) be saved.

Whatever time a shelter invests in temperament testing is time well spent. The risk and liability of not testing far outweigh any perceived lack of time.

CHAPTER 5

The AAP Baseline Tests Step by Step

How is the dog evaluated?

For each part of the test, the dog's possible responses fall into three categories: (A) dogs with lowest risk. i.e., dogs with the greatest potential to become successful pet dogs; (B) dogs at moderate risk for problematic, severely problematic, and aggressive behavior in the home; and (C) dogs at high risk for severely problematic behavior, including violence toward humans and other animals. The Assess-A-Pet Step by Step section in this manual gives a full range of possible responses for each procedure and ranks them into risk categories.

If the dog tests out as high risk in one part of the test, it is generally not safe for the tester to continue to the next part. For example, if the dog shows minimal or no sociability in the Sociability tests, it can be dangerous to proceed to the Teeth Exam. And if the dog reached his aggression threshold quickly during the Teeth Exam, he is unlikely to be safe to handle in other ways.

Unfortunately, at many shelters, staff, board members and volunteers unfamiliar with temperament testing and dubious of its predictive value often force testers to proceed with testing a dog until an overt aggressive display is elicited. In these cases, where a dog passes only one or none of the Sociability tests, it is best to proceed from the Sociability test directly to the tests for Resource Guarding, and from Resource Guarding to the Dog-Dog test. These are tests that can be done with a minimum of risk to the tester, but can sometimes clarify or reveal overt and/or dangerous aggression in the dog without putting the tester at great risk.

Only highly experienced testers should make the decision to proceed with the test after a dog exhibits an increased or high risk response, and only with other highly experienced dog people assisting.

No one should have to place himself in danger, or get threatened or bitten, in order to predict whether a dog will bite.

Scoring the responses

There are three categories of responses:

A = Low risk behaviors observed; most likely to be suitable as a pet

B = More risk behaviors observed; indicates an increased risk of serious behavior problems and aggression

C = High risk responses observed; aggression towards humans or other dogs/animals is probable, young children/elderly are at particular risk; possibility for human killings or dog killings

Note: The Sociability test is scored on a numerical basis (see page 33).

A responses: Dogs in this category are most likely to be suitable as pets, and/or as hobby sports participants; dogs scoring in this category have the highest aggression thresholds, and, along with a sociability score of 9 or higher, have the greatest likelihood for success in society.

B responses: Dogs in this category manifest an increasing risk for serious problem behaviors, and should be adopted out carefully, to adult-only homes where people have the time and inclination to learn about dog behavior and body language, and who are interested in training. Dogs in this category should be identified for behavior modification and training at the shelter. Dogs in this category benefit from learning skills while at the shelter, in particular learning to default to attention toward the handler (eye contact, attention, "watch me" exercises); basic cues such as sit, lie down, and stay/okay, plus a variety of tricks; and impulse control exercises.

Dogs in this category tend to have higher levels of predatory behaviors, and are hence harder to walk and exercise.

Dogs in this category are likely to have a longer than average length of stay in a shelter and a high risk for return, even multiple returns.

Dogs in this category are at greater risk for aggressive behaviors in the home, such as snapping at or biting family, guests, strangers, other dogs, etc. Adopters of dogs in this category must be aware of the need to compromise and make one or more serious to severe lifestyle modifications. These include but are not limited to:

- ❑ 100% management and training regime while out in public
- ❑ Limiting petting and interaction to one or two familiar people, and complete restrictions from strangers
- ❑ No hiking with the dog on or off leash
- ❑ Restricted outings with the dog in public
- ❑ The dog may be unable to be left alone

The "B response" dog can be viewed as questionable in terms of adoptability. This is a dog that should not be adopted out to the public for them to "figure out;" that is the responsibility of the shelter. In shelters with many adoptable dogs and few resources or adopters, a problematic/severely problematic dog might be euthanized in order to assure the best chance for adoption for all the behaviorally appropriate dogs that have a good chance for a successful placement.

For shelters with a training and behavior department and ample space and time, dogs with an increased risk of problematic and possibly some severe problematic behaviors may be targeted for further testing, behavior modification programs, training or fostering. Quality of life issues are paramount, and the mental and emotional needs of these difficult dogs should be assessed on a weekly basis to ensure humane conditions.

C responses: *Dogs in this category should be considered high risk for aggression toward humans or other dogs/animals; young children are at particular risk.* The dog is likely a danger to family and society, and/or other animals, and is unsuitable as a pet or working dog. If a C response dog is on the smaller side, he is likely to cause injuries and psychological and financial damage to humans and other animals; if medium-sized or larger, he is likely to get loose from his owner and maul or kill someone else's pet, or severely bite, maul or kill a person. This dog is at great risk of harming shelter staff and/or volunteers. Dogs with high-risk responses should immediately become unavailable to the public and volunteers. Shelters that euthanize will euthanize these dogs; shelters that do not euthanize may plan to kennel the dog permanently—but of course they will need to achieve and assure quality of life for these dogs *for the rest of their lives* in a shelter or in an on-site, regularly-inspected sanctuary.

> ### The adoption paradox
> The paradox in adopting out low-threshold (B/C Responses) dogs is that the people most capable and knowledgeable about how to possibly manage and live successfully with them are the very people who, when asked, state that while they loved their previous dog, and wouldn't have wanted not to have known him/her, *for their next dog, they would never do it again.* The potential adopter, listening to what adopting a low-threshold dog entails, cannot really imagine what life is truly like with a management-for-life, problematic dog. You have to have lived with one to truly know.

What does sociability look like?

All of the AAP tests involve observing the dog in question and making judgments about how the dog behaves in a number of circumstances. More experienced testers, especially ones with a good knowledge of behavior and body language, should be able to evaluate and score what they observe using the scoring charts included in the following sections for each of the tests. As I discuss in Chapter 7, being good at reading temperament means being able to read subtle body language. For less experienced testers, here is a listing of some of the responses of what you might observe and what they might indicate in terms of sociability and adoptability:

Sociable behaviors:

- ❏ Forehead smooth, ears back, eyes small, dog's eyes, head and spine are not in alignment, dog's tail is level or low
- ❏ Wide, sweeping wag or low tail wag
- ❏ Soft expression
- ❏ Dog will not be looking directly at your eyes without frequent blinking (more than once every two seconds)
- ❏ Eyes will be small, in particular with lower lids coming up to cover part of the eye
- ❏ Back of lips/commissures will be curled and pulled back
- ❏ Blinking will be more frequent than once every two seconds
- ❏ Comes readily and eagerly, little cajoling is needed
- ❏ Approaches unaligned (head, eyes and spine offset)
- ❏ Lowers the base of the tail the closer he comes to the tester
- ❏ Smooths out his forehead and puts his ears back/sideways
- ❏ Wags his tail low and wide-sweeping
- ❏ Dog grovels/crawls/approaches low to interact
- ❏ Shows a cashew/crescent shaped approach

Riskier behaviors:

- ❏ Hard expression
- ❏ Eyes are open and round
- ❏ Ears are erect or forward
- ❏ Sustained two seconds or longer direct eye contact
- ❏ Brow furrowed
- ❏ Infrequent blinking, less than once every two seconds

- ❑ Growling with barking
- ❑ Hackles up
- ❑ High arousal
- ❑ Consistently high tail
- ❑ Freeze in position
- ❑ Stiffening up, or remaining stiff
- ❑ Muscling up
- ❑ Muzzle bop, tap or punch
- ❑ Mouth on human
- ❑ Teeth on human

You may want to review some of the many good books or DVDs on the subject of canine body language, reactivity and aggression so that you will feel more comfortable making judgments about the behaviors you observe while conducting these tests. I have noted a few at the back of the book in the Recommended Reading and Viewing section.

Further observations that affect scoring

Additional red flags that increase risk:

- ❑ Dog weighs 40 pounds or more (increased risk if dog does have a bite event)
- ❑ Dog is powerful, muscular and athletic
- ❑ Dog pulls very hard when on regular leash/collar or slip lead (frequent lunge-aways, dog's head is frequently down and weight is frequently on his front end, etc.)
- ❑ Two or more known re-homings (including returns, incoming from another shelter where dog had a return, or passed along in the community, etc.)
- ❑ Dog requires limited volunteer access (possibly due to dog's strength or incident while at the shelter, etc.)
- ❑ When kenneled, dog lunges/charges/barks hard at passing dogs or humans
- ❑ Dog has a longer than average length of stay in the shelter
- ❑ Dog has developed a repetitive kennel behavior (spinning, route-tracing, pacing, triple rebound off side of kennel, etc.)
- ❑ Dog has a known history of serious problem behaviors
- ❑ Dog has a nipping/snapping/biting behavior history

Establishing a baseline

When scoring is completed, these following tests will give you a baseline idea of the dog's aggression thresholds. If the testing leaves the dog in a gray area category—low or no sociability, competitive but did not reach threshold on resources, prickly/stiff/testy with other dogs but not seeking harm—and there is not enough information about the dog to feel comfortable placing him on the adoption floor, nor is there basis for euthanasia, the additional tests can give you more information. If the shelter is a large, open-admission facility, with large numbers of dogs coming in daily, and fully assessing all the dogs is difficult, the base tests are an appropriate way to do behavioral triage upon arrival to fast-track the most adoptable dogs to the adoption floor, and safely take out the most dangerous.

In an ideal world, every shelter would fully assess all the dogs for which it is safe to do so.

Cage Presentation test step by step

Step One:

- ❏ Stand in front of the kennel, upright, facing frontal to the kennel. Look directly but neutrally at the dog's eyes.
- ❏ If or when the dog looks at you, count to five seconds while maintaining neutral, direct eye contact.

Step Two:

- ❏ Turn sideways, squat down, and smile, cajole and baby talk to the dog. Continue for five seconds.

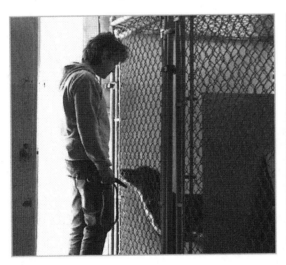

Step One

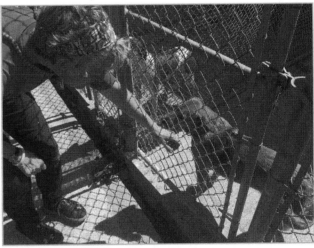

Step Two

Cage Presentation test responses and scoring

Note: Score A for adoptable; B for increased risk of aggression; C for high risk of aggression.

Score	Responses	Step 1	Step 2	Notes
A	Dog has low, wide, sweeping wag or circular wag at front of kennel			
A	Dog's spine is consistently curved or crescent-shaped at front of kennel			
A	Dog grovels/crawls/ approaches low to interact			
A	Dog's rear end is lower than front end at least half the time			
A	Dog carries tail level or low consistently			
A	Dog keeps eyes, head, spine unaligned during all interactions			
B	Dog's tail is carried high consistently			
B	Hackles up			
B	Dog does not approach front of kennel			
B	Dog's feet move hardly or not at all			
B	Dog's eyes, head and spine are aligned consistently while dog orients to tester			

Score	Responses	Step 1	Step 2	Notes
B	Dog barks or growls but stops within three seconds			
B	Dog consistently remains in back of kennel, whites of eyes show, stiff body			
B	Dog barks			
B	Dog growls			
B	High arousal, consistently high tail; no interaction			
C	Dog engages in repetitive behavior (leaping up and down, rebounding off kennel wall, spinning, pacing, etc.)			
C	Growling, snarling			
C	Growling with barking			
C	Dog at front of kennel lunging, barking, snapping, trying to bite			

If the dog scores mostly A responses with two or fewer B responses in this test, proceed with Sociability testing. You will need to get the dog out of the kennel to begin Sociability testing.

Getting the dog out of the kennel

To do this:

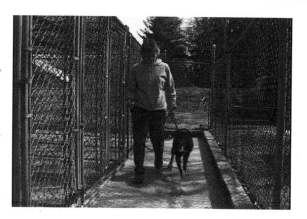

- ❑ Approach the dog in the kennel from a sideways, standing, neutral position.

- ❑ Have your leash ready to loop over the dog's head.

- ❑ Open the kennel door a crack, and slip your leash in.

- ❑ Leash the dog from a sideways, neutral position.

- ❑ Let the dog walk into the noose and once he is noosed, open the kennel door and let him exit.

- ❑ Young dogs (under a year) that have not been on leash before or won't walk at all on a leash, and have had no behavioral concerns, can be safely carried to the testing area. This excludes non-social and/or defensive balking dogs. Always use caution when lifting a dog.

- ❑ Keep your weight on both feet, with knees relaxed, and feet far enough apart to maintain your stability.

- ❑ Remember to keep a constant, steady tension on the leash.

Leash handling tips:

- ◻ Avoid yanking or pulling sharply on the leash at any time. Keep a constant, light tension on the leash.

- ◻ For shy or nervous dogs, the tester may kneel down from outside the kennel and cajole and encourage the dog forward. Try not to corner a nervous dog to get him out.

Sociability Test step-by-step

The Sociability test is comprised of four sub-tests. These tests serve an important role in evaluating a dog, and I believe Sociability is the single most important test in Assess-A-Pet. A dog with low or no sociability poses a much greater risk for the tester; low sociability has been associated with lowered aggression thresholds and the greater likelihood of problem behaviors in the home, and in my experience and with anecdotal evidence, dogs with low or no sociability are likely to have a longer length of stay in the kennels.

Please note: In many higher crime area shelters, the majority of dogs are likely to have low or no sociability. In shelters where the majority of the population of dogs have low or no sociability, this can inadvertently become the "new normal" for testers, and may cause a loosening and lowering of adoption criteria.

Don't exercise the dog before the test

If the dog has held his bladder/bowels and needs to potty, this should be done prior to testing, i.e., take the dog to potty and then return him to his kennel, test a different dog, and return to the original dog so that you can take a dog straight from the kennel to the testing room. Why is it important to bring the dog straight into the testing room without pottying or exercising the dog first? It is in the dog's best interest to come directly into the testing room and start the Sociability tests. Pottying, walking and exercising can all increase arousal and frustration, and cause the dog to take longer to settle and orient/show sociability toward the tester.

It is in the dog's best interest to not allow exploration of the room, on or off leash. This can only serve to distract the dog, to encourage him to be engaged by things in the environment other than the tester. It serves to encourage social contact and orientation to bring the dog directly in on a restricted leash and start the testing.

Step One: Stand and ignore for 60 seconds

1. Enter the testing room and stop. If at all possible, place yourself with your back against a wall.

> ### Why lean against a wall?
>
> This is not just to put the tester in a safer, more stable position (cannot be knocked backwards) but also to help limit the dog to 180 degrees in front of the tester—offering the dog potentially a better chance at showing sociability/orienting to the tester.

2. Observation of sociability begins at this point.

3. Allow the dog about 4 feet of leash.

4. Begin timing 60 seconds.

5. Ignore the dog—remain firmly planted, but relaxed. Be receptive if the dog makes sociable contact by remaining relaxed and neutral, leaning over on one hip if possible. Feel free to smile at the dog. Don't talk to the dog or initiate an interaction, but don't stiffen or reject the dog. If the dog jumps up, don't discourage him. If the dog is jumping hard at you, or in an aggressive way, turn your body away.

6. This part of the test ends at 60 seconds.

> ### Can this test be done off leash?
>
> With puppies 4 months and under, or toy-sized dog that has not previously been on leash, or toy dogs showing no red flag behaviors during Cage Presentation and with no history of problematic or risky behaviors, the Sociability tests can be done off leash, while the tester kneels or squats, with an ex-pen enclosing them.

Step Two: Three back strokes

1. Gather up the leash.

2. Place yourself so that the dog is somewhat in front of you, in profile.

3. Bend down and stroke the dog slowly and deeply, starting at the back of the neck and continuing down to the base of the tail. Each stroke should last about one and a half seconds.

4. Stand upright and pause for one full second between each stroke.

5. Repeat for a total of three strokes.

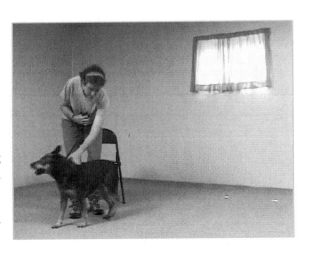

Keep safe while stroking:

- The hand closest to the dog's head should have the gathered portion of the leash, so the tester ends up with a short enough leash to be close to the dog's neck but just out of range of the mouth if the dog reaches up.

- When you begin stroking, step back one step, to keep your body just out of reach, and extend and straighten the elbow of the arm holding the leash. This serves to keep you in the best defensive position if the dog should become aggressive.

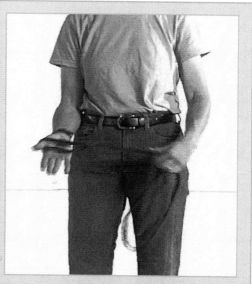

Testing puppies

With puppies four months and younger, or toy dogs with no problematic behaviors, the tester may kneel or sit on the floor.

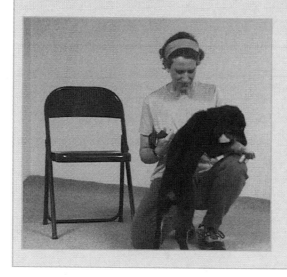
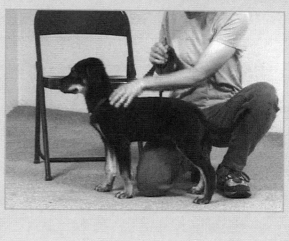

Step Three: Sit in a chair

1. Allow the dog about 4 feet of leash.

2. Sit in a chair without saying anything. Gather the leash up as you sit, so that as the dog approaches you still have no tension or slack in the leash.

3. Ignore the dog for a count of five seconds.

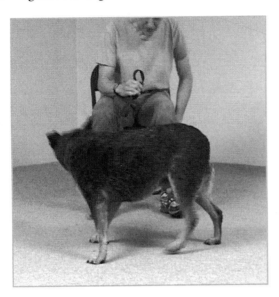 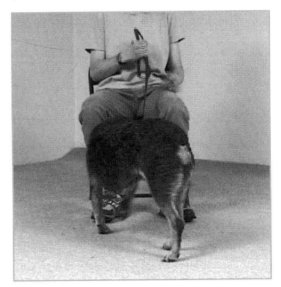

If the dog invades your space or comes too close to your face:

- If the dog comes up toward the tester's face, the tester can keep one hand, palm facing outward toward dog, back of hand touching the tester, as a barrier/protection for tester's face and neck. Do not push or shove the dog.

- If at any point you feel uncomfortable or threatened, stand up and let gravity displace the dog off of you.

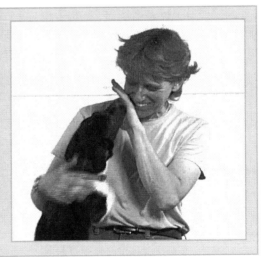

Step Four: 20 seconds of affection

1. While sitting in the chair, place your hands, palms down with the backs of your facing up on your lap. While tapping your thighs, cajole and call and begin sweet-talking to the dog.

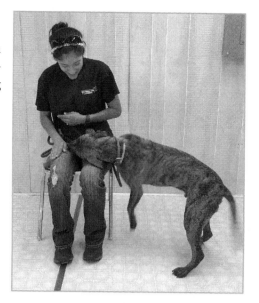

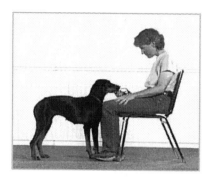

2. Begin timing 20 seconds.

3. Alternate between cajoling and petting the dog every two seconds; use sing-songy verbal banter, praise, smooching sounds, etc. and smile.

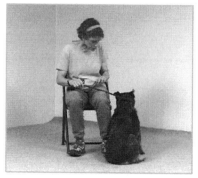 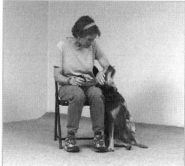 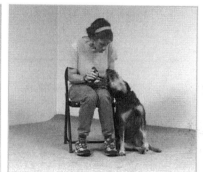

4. After 20 seconds, stop the test.

Safety and scoring tips for Sociability testing

The alternating cajoling and petting is to see if the dog is remaining on his own/getting sociability points for petting or only getting petted because the tester has reached out and is petting him. This facilitates scoring.

If the dog approaches, gather the leash to remain in the safest possible position. One hand will have the leash in it gathered almost completely.

Sociability test responses and scoring

Sociability gets scored differently than the other tests. The dog is given a numeric score in addition to the ABC system used in the other AAP tests. During each of the four Sociability sub-tests, the dog earns one point for every two second block of sustained, physical contact while orienting to the tester. There are three exclusions: Sniffing, Mounting and Biting (biting is defined as any teeth contact with tester's skin or clothes) which means that even if the dog is oriented to the tester, making physical contact, but is at the same time sniffing the tester's clothes, the counting stops and resumes again only after the dog stops sniffing (as long as the dog maintains physical contact while orienting toward the tester). The numeric score is accumulated during each of the four sub-tests based purely on sustained physical contact, while the A, B, C scoring adds observations based on the manner in which the dog orients himself to the tester and what he looks like doing so. The score is calculated in the following four steps:

1. As soon as the dog makes physical contact while orienting to the tester, begin counting ("one Mississippi, two Mississippi") etc.

2. For every two second block of sustained physical contact, give the dog one point (e.g., the dog nuzzles the tester's hand for two full seconds = 1 point; if the dog jumps up on the tester and keeps his paws up and touching for 7 seconds, the dog gets 3 points, etc.).

3. If the dog makes sustained physical contact but is not orienting toward the tester (leans against the tester's leg sideways, or jumps on tester's lap from side and faces away from tester, for example), he receives no points.

4. Points earned during each of the four Sociability sub-tests are added together to form the final score—for example, two points earned during Sit in A Chair are added to the ten points the dog earns during the 20 Seconds of Affection, for a final score of 12.

Scoring is as follows:

9 and higher = Least risky behaviors; most likely to be suitable as pet

5 to 8 = Increasing risk for problem behaviors

0 to 4 = Increasing risk for problem behaviors, increasing risk for aggression and more severe aggression

Other aspects of the Sociability tests (see the following test response charts) are scored A, B or C and serve as a further guide to help you score the four tests. Refer back to the above heading "What does sociability look like" as another way to help train your eye in the nuances of sociable contact.

While this dog is making physical contact with the taster, he is not orienting toward the tester and is therefore not earning sociability points.

Dogs that score 9 and higher: These are dogs with medium and high sociability, and are more likely to make suitable pets; dogs scoring here and scoring in A responses in the tests are suitable for Level One, Two and Three adopters; dogs with these scores in sociability and B responses in other tests (resource guarding or dog-dog testing) may make successful pets with careful placement with Level Three adopters or professional trainers and behaviorists in carefully selected environments.

Dogs that score 5 through 8: Dog with these scores and A categories in all other tests may make suitable pets with Level Two or Three adopters; dogs with these sociability scores and score mostly B in other tests are more risky, usually have a longer than average length of stay, should not be around young children; dogs with these sociability scores and mostly C scores in other tests are significantly more risky, and both B and C scores have a higher risk of return/multiple returns.

Dogs that score 0 through 4: These dogs have low or no sociability and are considered high-risk placements. Dogs with these scores and A categories in all other tests, are at increased length of stay, should not be around young children, have a higher risk of returns/multiple returns. Dogs scoring B and C in other tests are at increased risk of aggression problem behaviors/aggression while at the shelter, and significantly more risky—if not downright dangerous.

The body language check list on pages 22-23 ultimately trumps the numerical scoring, as there are times when a dog will score sociability points with physical contact that does not meet the A or B category and thus indicates a risky dog.

Note: Behaviors are listed in increasing order of risk in each category. So the first behavior is less risky than the last behavior.

Sociability test responses and scoring

Score	Responses	Step 1	Step 2	Step 3	Step 4	Notes/ Observations
A	Dog has low, wide sweeping wag or circular wag					
A	Dog grovels/ crawls/approaches low to interact					
A	Dog carries tail level or low consistently					
A	Dog carries tail level or just above level consistently					
A	Dog's tail is carried high but lowers during three strokes and 20 Seconds of Affection					
B	Dog's tail is high/ remains high, or raises higher than plane of dog's back during interaction					
B	Three or more leash bops or nose bops					
B	Two or more jump with clasps					
B	Two or more pounce offs					

Score	Responses	Step 1	Step 2	Step 3	Step 4	Notes/ Observations
B	More than three shoulder swipes/ or two shoulder stances					
B	Two or more anal swipe/anal plants					
B	Face diving (two or more)					
B	Head whip					
B	Dog puts mouth on tester					
C	Dog turns to look directly at tester— direct eye contact, blinking less than once every two seconds					
C	More than three lunge-aways					
C	Dog's feet move hardly or not at all					
C	Dog's eyes, head and spine are aligned consistently while dog orients to tester					
C	Mounts					
C	High arousal, consistently high tail					
C	Dog begins high-energy barking					
C	Dog air snaps, clacks teeth while jumping					
C	Dog puts mouth on tester, bears down, pressure					

Score	Responses	Step 1	Step 2	Step 3	Step 4	Notes/ Observations
C	Freeze/stiffening/ muscling up					
C	Dog growls					
C	Dog snaps/ attempts to bite/ bites					

Resource Guarding tests step by step

The following tests look at aggression thresholds for guarding valued resources. While the items used to test are a cloth toy, a pig's ear or similar edible chewable toy, and the food bowl, dogs placed into homes with low thresholds for resource guarding are as or more likely to guard owners, territory, crates/cars, and if the adopter has another dog, develop dog-dog aggression problems (usually owner guarding).

Testing using the items in this section of assessing aggression thresholds is not just about looking for a direct correlation between test responses to the food bowl and chewable bones and then comparable food and bone guarding behaviors post-adoption. It is, like all the other tests, a test for aggression thresholds in the pet dog. Test results that indicate lower thresholds in one or more categories most often predict highly problematic/ severe behavior problems in the home (as well as, of course, an increased likelihood of food, bone and toy guarding). In my experience, the dog most likely to have severe separation anxiety in the home is the low/non-sociable, resource-guarding dog. This may be because there is often an anxiety component to the aggressive dog, and thus he becomes extra anxious when alone, or maybe the resource guarding dog feels he must guard the territory/home/objects/owners, and when he is left alone, he falls apart because he does not really know what to do with all his "stuff."

It is here in the resource guarding tests that the need for a revision from the original AAP was most critical. With shelters testing larger and more athletic dogs, and more and more non-sociable dogs, the original procedures for testing resource guarding have become dangerous. While holding the dog on leash for testing was appropriate and safe enough in the past, the dogs of today are just too large, muscular and overall more dangerous, so dogs today should be tethered during the resource guarding tests.

A secure eye bolt that is bolted to the floor or low on a wall is the safest way to secure a dog. The dog should be clipped to the eye bolt with a leash that won't slip over his head. Use a consistent length of tether for all dogs.

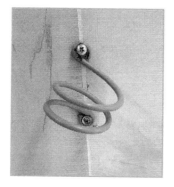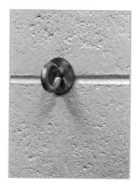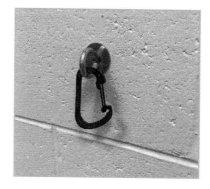

Examples of tethers.

If the dog shows little or no interest in the toy, pig's ear or food bowl used in these tests, find similar items of greater value until the dog becomes interested. Continue to retest until the dog shows interest. It is valid to increase the value of these items, or increase palatability (canned cat food, all canned food and no dry, etc.) in order to test the dog. It is the perceived value of each item for the dog that matters, not the actual item. If a dog is not interested in a testing item, the dog will need a retest before making him available for adoption. An inconclusive test because of lack of interest is not necessarily an indication of a safe dog.

Note: For safety, the tests for guarding require the use of an Assess-A-Hand (AAH).

The procedures for the resource guarding tests are very carefully laid out in a particular order, and it has been my experience that the earlier on in the process the dog hits an aggression threshold (freeze, growl, snarl, snap, bite), the more serious the level of aggression.

The step with the hesitant communication is critical, as this mimics the communication used by inexperienced owners, children and new adopters who don't yet know their dog.

Toy test step by step

Step One:

1. Take a cloth toy (rope toy, fleece doll, etc.) in one hand, and gather up the leash with the other hand, allowing about 3 feet of slack.

2. Entice the dog with the toy by dragging it on the floor in front of the dog, just out of reach, turning in a circle in the direction of the hand with the toy.

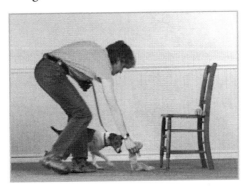 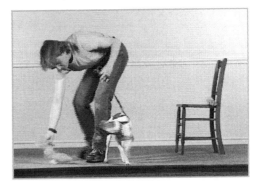

3. After at least one rotation, toss the toy about 4 or 5 feet away and give the dog slack to go to the toy.

Handling techniques to remember:

- If the dog is leashed rather than tethered, be sure to gather up slack in the leash as you approach so that there is no excess.

- If the Assess-A-Hand is in your right hand, keep the dog on your left side and the leash in your left hand, and vice versa.

- Always keep the Assess-A-Hand between you and the dog while you interact with the dog so that you can both control the dog with the leash/tether and use the Assess-A-Hand as a buffer from an aggressive dog.

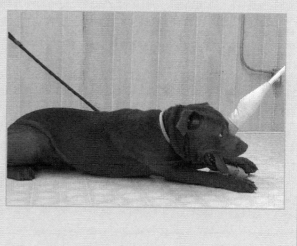

Step Two (do the following whether or not the dog is interested in the toy):

1. Give the dog a few seconds to become more interested in the toy. End by letting the dog have the toy and ignoring him until he settles down with the toy.

2. Hold the Assess-A-Hand behind your back so the dog doesn't see it before you use it.

3. Take one deliberate step toward the toy with one foot, then bring the other foot flush and stand neutrally. End up approximately 12 inches from the toy.

4. With the AAH, stroke the dog along his back and praise gently.

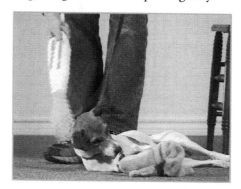

5. Pause, stand back up, then pat the dog gently on his head with the AAH and praise gently.

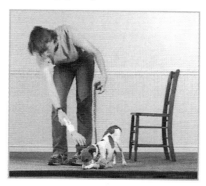

6.   Pause, stand back up, and then bring the AAH slowly down to the dog's mouth and the toy, and when within an inch of the toy, draw back suddenly as if you think the dog is going to bite. Repeat this for a total of three times.

7.   Finally, bring the back of the AAH all the way to the side of the dog's muzzle, and gently apply steady pressure to push the dog's muzzle away from the toy. Continue applying pressure for a few seconds and stop. Repeat once more for a total of two times.

No interest in toy?
Many dogs do not show an interest in the toy. This does not usually indicate a problem or need for retesting as long as there are no indications of guarding of the pig's ear or food bowl in the next two tests.

Resource Guarding Toy test responses and scoring

Note: All responses are to be considered more risky with sociability scores of 5 or less.

Note: Score A for adoptable; B for increased risk of aggression; C for high risk of aggression.

Score	Responses	Step 1	Step 2	Notes/Comments
A	Dog ignores toy and offers sociability			
A	Dog ignores toy			
A	Dog appears unfamiliar with toys/won't approach or engage, or backs away from toy			
A	Dog engages toy with low arousal/interest			
A	Dog engages toy with low or medium arousal, loses interest within five seconds			
A	Dog engages toy but disengages when tester approaches			
A	Dog looks from toy to tester and back to toy again			

Score	Responses	Step 1	Step 2	Notes/Comments
A	Dog shows whites of eyes/whale eye (no freezing or pausing or stiffening)			
A	Dog increases speed and intensity as test progresses			
A	Shoulder block			
B	Dog's tail raises higher over back			
B	Dog snatches resource and turns back on tester or pulls hard to a different location			
B	Dog drops toy or leaves toy and pounces with front paws hard against tester, rebounds off tester when tester faces or approaches toy			
B	Dog hovers or briefly freezes, less than one second			
C	Dog hovers or freezes, one second or longer			
C	Dog freezes/stiffens			
C	Dog snarls			
C	Dog growls			
C	Dog snaps			
C	Dog bites Assess-A-Hand			
C	Dog ignores Assess-A-Hand and tries to bite (or successfully bites) tester			

Pig's Ear test step by step

Preparation

1.   Place a blanket or towel on the floor in the testing area.

2.   Tether the dog to the tether point.

Step One: Give the dog the pig's ear:

1.   Begin by holding the Assess-A-Hand hidden behind your back, so you don't advertise it to the dog before testing begins.

2.   Give the dog a pig's ear or, if he won't take it from you, let the dog watch you toss it onto the blanket for him.

3.   Allow the dog to take the pig's ear (hopefully) to the blanket, or lie down where he is.

Step Two: Giant, deliberate step

1.   If the dog does show interest, try to wait for the dog to really settle, and put the pig's ear between his front paws and hopefully he starts using his back molars to chew it.

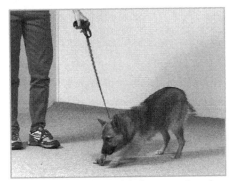

Wait for the dog to lie down and settle.

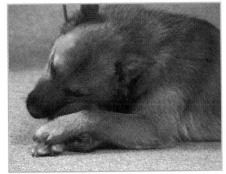

Wait for the dog to start using his back molars to chew before starting the assessment.

2.   Keep the Assess-A-Hand hidden behind your back.

3.   Whether or not the dog engages, take one deliberate, giant step up to the resource, planting one foot and bringing the other foot up flush, ending up within 12 inches of the resource. Observe the dog.

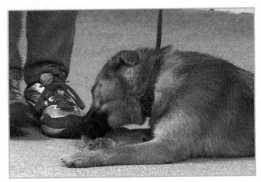
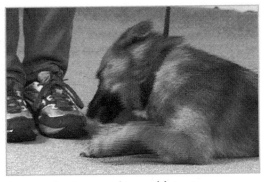

Take one deliberate, giant step up to the resource, planting one foot and bringing the other foot up flush, ending up within 12 inches of the resource.

Step Three: Stroke dog's back and praise

1. Take a step back, toward the dog's side/rear, if you can, so that you end up about one to two feet away from the dog, facing a similar direction

2. With the AAH, stroke the dog along its back and praise gently, "Are you a good dog? What a good dog..." for a total of two slow strokes.

Step Four: Stroke dog's head and praise

1. Withdraw and stand back up, and then, with the AAH, stroke and pat the top of the dog's head and praise gently, "Are you a good dog? What a gooooood dog!"

2. Do this for the time it takes you to say the phrases above.

Step Five: Three hesitant approaches/retreats

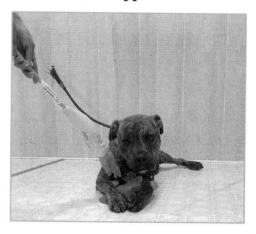 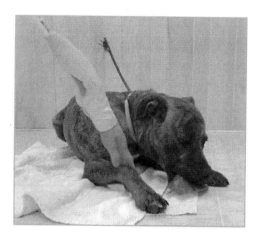

1. Stand back up, and approaching with the AAH bring the hand slowly down toward the resource, until you are almost touching it, and then, at the last minute, pull back suddenly, as if you thought the dog was about to bite.

2. Repeat this hesitant communication for a total of three approaches/retreats.

3. Try to time the retreats so that if the dog pauses, or freezes for a moment, that's when you retreat.

Step Six: Gentle steady pressure/push away

1. Finally, bring the back of the AAH all the way to the side of the dog's muzzle, and apply gentle-but-steady pressure to push the dog away from the pig's ear. Continue applying pressure for two full seconds and then withdraw. Repeat once more.

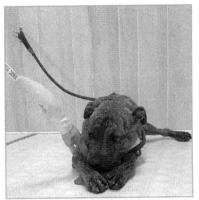 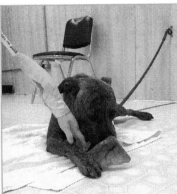

Apply gentle-but-steady pressure to push the dog away from the pig's ear.

Safety tips for the Pig's Ear test

- □ If leashed, be sure to gather up the slack as you approach the dog, always remaining in the best position for defensive handling.

- □ If leashed and if the AAH is in your right hand, keep the dog on your left side and the leash in your left hand and vice versa.

- □ If leashed, always keep the AAH between you and the dog while you interact so you can use the AAH as a buffer from harm.

- □ Stand up straight, bring the Assess-A-Hand behind your back, and pause briefly between each step before continuing.

- □ If the dog is uninterested in the pig's ear, you can try other valued, slow-chewing bones like Greenies, a peanut-butter-stuffed Kong, a beef basted marrow bone, etc.

- □ If the dog is uninterested in any of these chewable items, the dog is not considered safe. All dogs should be tested for their thresholds when chewing a valuable item other than their food.

Pig's Ear test responses and scoring

Note: All responses are considered more risky with sociability scores of 5 or less.

Note: Score A for adoptable; B for increased risk of aggression; C for high risk of aggression.

Score	Responses	Steps 1-4	Step 5-6	Notes/Comments
A	Dog chews item and begins wide wagging when tester approaches			
A	Dog shows mild/moderate interest in chewing; wags hard or harder when tester makes contact			
A	Dog shows mild/moderate interest in chewing; disengages briefly to look at tester while wagging			
A	Dog is playful with resource—tosses it in air, and/or takes resource closer to tester to chew			
A	Dog chews item and never increases in speed or intensity throughout the test			
A	Dog engages but disengages when tester approaches and offers sociability in a position not blocking access to resource			
A	Dog looks from resource to tester and back to resource again			

Score	Responses	Steps 1-4	Step 5-6	Notes/Comments
A	Dog shows whites of eyes/whale eye			
A	Dog shows more interest in the resource after the tester either steps toward or engages in testing			
A	Shoulder block			
A	Dog increases speed and intensity as test progresses/ tester gets closer			
B	Dog's tail raises higher over back			
B	Dog snatches resource and turns back on tester or pulls hard to a different location			
B	Dog rubs shoulder on toy			
B	Dog drops toy or leaves pigs ear and pounces with front paws hard against tester, rebounds off tester when tester faces or approaches pigs ear			
B	Dog hovers or briefly freezes, less than one second			
C	Dog hovers or freezes one second or longer			
C	Dog freezes/stiffens			

Score	Responses	Steps 1-4	Step 5-6	Notes/Comments
C	Dog snarls			
C	Dog growls			
C	Dog snaps			
C	Dog bites Assess-A-Hand			
C	Dog skirts around Assess-A-Hand and tries to bite (or successfully bites) tester			

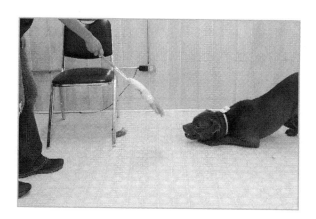

Dog snarls.

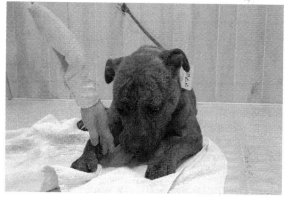

Dog hovers or freezes one second or longer.

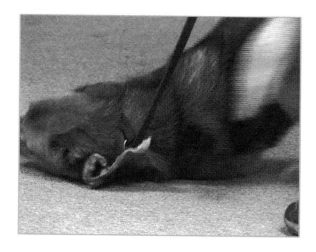

Dog rubs shoulder on toy.

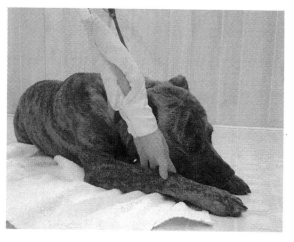

Dog freezes for more than one second.

Scoring notes

❑ The earlier in the sequence the dog hits an aggression threshold (freeze is the first behavior indicating the dog has hit threshold), the more serious the aggression.

❑ Dogs with high sociability that do small freezes, short snarls, short growls, or slow-motion snaps are less risky than dogs with low or no sociability and the same behaviors.

Resource Guarding: Food Bowl test

To begin the test, fill a large food bowl with a mixture of dry kibble and wet food. Mix well; moisten with water if necessary to distribute gravy; make sure food reaches almost to top.

Step One: Give the dog the food bowl

Place bowl on floor and stand back a step.

Step Two: Giant, deliberate step

1. Wait for the dog to start eating.

2. Keep the Assess-A-Hand hidden behind your back.

3. Whether or not the dog engages, take one deliberate, giant step up to the food bowl, planting one foot and bringing the other foot up flush, ending up within 12 inches of the resource. Observe the dog.

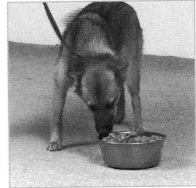

Make sure food reaches almost to the top of the bowl.

Step Three: Stroke dog's back and praise

1. Take a step toward the dog's side/rear, if you can, so that you end up about one to two feet away from the dog, facing a similar direction.

2. If you have to do the test from directly in front of the dog, proceed.

3. With the Assess-A-Hand, stroke the dog along his back and praise gently, "Are you a good dog? What a good dog…" for a total of two slow strokes.

4. Do this for the full time it takes you to say the phrases above.

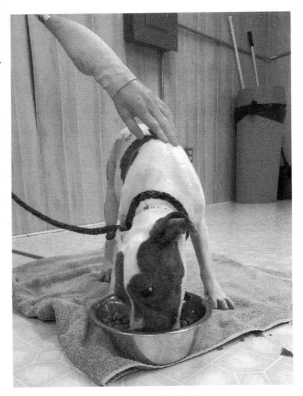

Stroke the dog along his back and praise.

Step Four: Three hesitant approaches/retreats

1. Stand back up, and approaching with the Assess-A-Hand bring the hand slowly down toward the food bowl, until you are almost touching it, and then, at the last minute, pull back suddenly, as if you thought the dog was about to bite.

2. Repeat this hesitant communication for a total of three approaches/retreats.

3. Try to time the retreats so that if the dog pauses, or freezes for a moment, that's when you retreat.

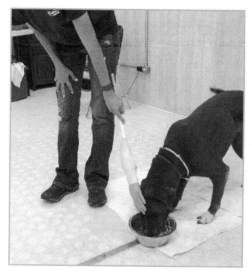 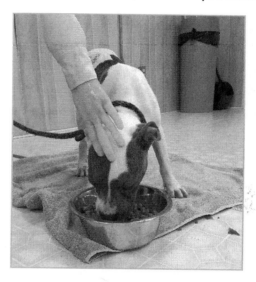

With the Assess-A-Hand, stroke and pat the top of the dog's head and praise gently, "Are you a good dog? What a gooooood dog!"

Step Five: Gentle steady pressure/push away

Finally, bring the back of the Assess-A-Hand all the way to the side of the dog's muzzle, and apply gentle-but-steady pressure to push the dog away from the food bowl. Continue applying pressure for two full seconds and then withdraw. Repeat once more.

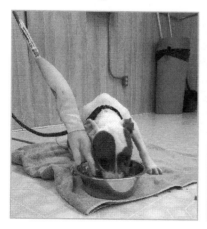 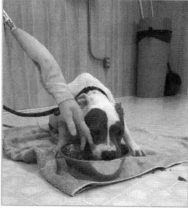 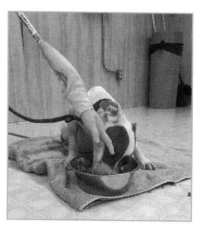

Apply gentle-but-steady pressure to push the dog away from the food bowl.

Food Bowl test responses and scoring

Note: All responses are considered more risky with sociability scores of 5 or less.

Note: Score A for adoptable; B for increased risk of aggression; C for high risk of aggression.

Score	Responses	Step 1	Step 2	Step 3	Step 4	Step 5	Notes
A	Dog wide wags while eating when tester touches or approaches						
A	Dog eats food at same rate during entire test						
A	Dog wide wags and looks up, ears go back, eyes squint, forehead relaxes and then goes back to eating						
A	Dog wide wags harder during back strokes and head pats						
A	Dog moves muzzle closer to tester's side of bowl when tester approaches/ touches						
A	Dog looks from food bowl to tester and back to food bowl again						

Score	Responses	Step 1	Step 2	Step 3	Step 4	Step 5	Notes
A	Dog shows whites of eyes/whale eye						
A	Dog increases speed and intensity as test progresses						
A	Shoulder block						
B	Dog's tail raises higher over back						
B	Dog hovers or briefly freezes, less than one second						
B	Dog hovers or freezes one second or longer						
B	Dog freezes/ stiffens						
C	Dog snarls						
C	Dog growls						
C	Dog snaps						
C	Dog bites Assess-A-Hand						
C	Dog skirts around Assess-A-Hand and tries to bites (or successfully bites) tester						

Safety tips and notes for Food Bowl test

- If the dog shows little or no interest in the food, or he picks out the chunks, remove the bowl and try mixing in something of higher value or start fresh with a new bowl of higher value food, perhaps all wet.

- Always make sure you know where the edge of the dog's tether extends, and how far you are from the dog.

- Stand up straight, bring the Assess-A-Hand behind your back, and pause briefly between each step before continuing.

- The bowl must be full enough at all times during testing so that the dog can eat and still have enough food in the bowl to compete for it if approached. If the bowl has too little food in it, many food-aggressive dogs will simply gobble the food before you can finish the test, and you can miss crucial responses.

Notes

- ❑ The earlier in the sequence the dog hits an aggression threshold, the more serious the aggression.

- ❑ Dogs with high sociability that do small freezes, short snarls, short growls, or slow-motion snaps are less risky than dogs with low or no sociability and the same behaviors.

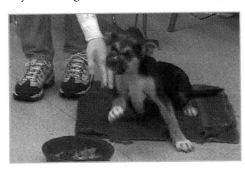 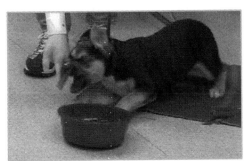

Aggression in young puppies is more concerning than aggression in adolescents or older dogs.

Dog-Dog testing step by step

Step One: 45 seconds of distance

1. Bring the dog into the testing area.

2. Bring in a familiar dog or neutral dog.

3. Both dogs remain on leash, at least 8 feet apart, but no more than 50 feet apart. Allow dogs to see each other, but not interact.

4. Restrain the dogs at this distance for 45 seconds.

5. If the leash is tight and the dog straining, the tester should just plant his feet and hold.

6. As long as the responses of the dogs during the restraint contain no red flags, proceed to the next step.

Step Two: Approach

1. Have each handler approach each other, step-by-step, re-evaluating behaviors and responses at each step.

2. If there are any concerns, the neutral dog should leave and be replaced with a stuffed dog. (Proceed to Page 55 and see Testing Procedures for the Stuffed Dog.)

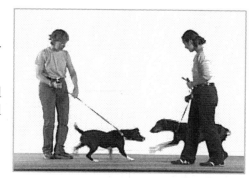

Step Three: Nose-to-nose

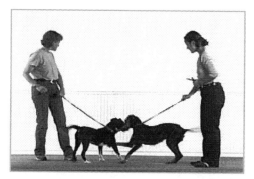

1. The two real dogs should approach each other until they are nose to nose. The handlers' leashes should still be taut, so there is complete control of distance between dogs (in case dogs need to be pulled apart suddenly).

2. Observe dogs while they are nose-to-nose for two seconds. Proceed to the next step only if there are no concerns.

The handlers' leashes should still be taut, so there is complete control of distance between dogs (in case dogs need to be pulled apart suddenly).

Step Four: Loose leash interactions

Handlers will loosen leashes and let the dogs interact; handlers should be prepared to "maypole" around the dogs, as the dogs will likely circle, and the handlers should try to stay a step ahead of the dogs to avoid tangling of leashes.

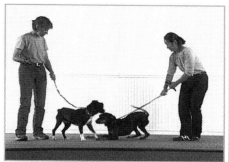
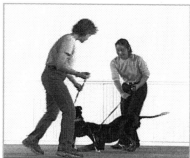
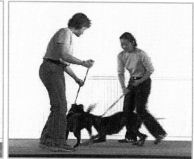

Dog-Dog test responses and scoring

Note: All responses are considered more risky with sociability scores of 5 or less.

Note: Score A for adoptable; B for increased risk of aggression; C for high risk of aggression.

Score	Responses	Step 1	Step 2	Step 3	Step 4	Notes
A	Dog looks away from other dog and makes sociable eye contact with tester more than once					
A	Dog changes position: shifts, turns from other dog to other points in room or toward tester multiple times					
A	Dog's ears shift positions multiple times in each procedure					
A	Dog spends over 50% of time looking at people or things other than the dog					
A	Base of dog's tail moves many times during each procedure—up, down, level, low, wide wag, no wag, wags a little					
A	Dog's eyes, head and spine are unaligned most of the time					
A	Dog's body weight is underneath him for most of the interactions—neither forward nor back					
A	Dog shifts from standing, to turning, to sitting, to bowing, to lying down multiple times					

Score	Responses	Step 1	Step 2	Step 3	Step 4	Notes
B	Dog shoulder swipes handler					
B	Dog looks at/orients toward/stares at other dog for more than 50% of the time					
B	Dog's tail raises higher over back					
B	Dog's tail remains high for most of procedures					
B	Dog raises wide hackles along back					
B	Dog raises a thin line of hackles between shoulders or along back of neck					
B	Dog mounts					
B	Dog remains still and doesn't move feet for many seconds at a time while staring at other dog					
B	Dog's eyes, head and spine are aligned more than 50% of the time					
B/C	Dog begins to whine and/or tremble					
B/C	Dog's arousal levels (breathing rate, rate of panting, excitability, etc.) rise steadily throughout test					
B/C	Dog freezes/stiffens					
B/C	Dog snarls					
B/C	Dog growls					

Score	Responses	Step 1	Step 2	Step 3	Step 4	Notes
B/C	Dog snaps					
B/C	Dog is pulling forward, or straining hard on leash toward the other dog more than 50% of the time					
B/C	Dog spends more than 50% of the time on his hind legs					
C	Dog makes hard physical contact, crashes into the other dog and/or pummels him with no communication					
C	Dog head whips (extreme handler risk)					
C	Dog tries to bite other dog					
C	Dog whips head and tries to bite handler					

The combination "B/C" responses are due to the inconsistent nature of the behaviors of the other dog. Some aggressive displays are warranted if the other dog is behaving in an intrusive, bullying or aggressive manner.

If you have to use a fake stuffed dog

A stuffed dog replaces the real, live dog after the first step of the test (45 seconds of restraint at a distance), or at anytime during testing, if the dog you are testing is deemed too risky to approach using the real dog. When using a stuffed dog, try to have a standing, large-breed dog. I recommend placing a used dog collar on the stuffed one, complete with jingling tags. Wherever the real dog left the testing room, the stuffed dog should appear from that exit.

Step One

1. Bring in the stuffed dog from wherever you took away the real dog.

2. Restrain both dogs (the real dog you are testing and the stuffed dog) at a distance for 45 seconds. Observe the dog.

3. Allow the real dog to go to the stuffed dog as fast as he wants, so run behind him if you need to. When he gets to the fake dog, allow him a loose leash to do whatever he wants. Observe the dog.

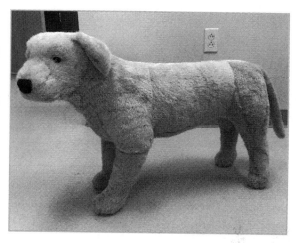

Fake stuffed dog profile.

Step Two

1. After the real dog has had a chance to behave how he wants once he gets to the stuffed one, have your helper maneuver the stuffed dog so that he turns and confronts the real dog by turning and facing him directly. Observe the dog.

2. Have your helper make the fake dog place his chin onto the shoulders of the real dog. Observe the dog.

Step Three

Lastly, have the helper make the fake dog turn his back on the real dog, and pull the fake dog suddenly away and see if the real dog wants to give chase.

Safety tips and notes

If one dog gets his foot caught over the leash, or the leashes become tangled, the tester should reach down toward the dog's collar and grab the base of the leash, dropping the handle end while quickly pulling the leash up from the base. Do not pick up the dog's foot or reach underneath the dog, as this is risky.

Stuffed Dog test responses and scoring

Note: Score A for adoptable; B for increased risk of aggression; C for high risk of aggression.

Score	Responses	Step 1	Step 2	Step 3	Notes
B	Dog looks at/orients toward/stares at other dog for more than 50% of the time				
B	Dog's tail raises higher over back				
B	Dog's tail remains high for most of procedures				
B	Dog stiffens/freezes				
C	Dog's arousal level (breathing rate, rate of panting, excitability, etc.) rises steadily or spikes				
C	Dog whines and/or trembles				
C	Dog rushes over to stuffed dog and circles and/or sniffs				
C	Dog mounts, with or without hackles raised				
C	Dog rushes over to stuffed dog and bites/knocks down without sniffing or stopping first				
C	Dog bites stuffed dog				
C	Dog bites and shakes stuffed dog				
C	Dog bites and yanks stuffed dog to ground				
C	Dog whips head and tries to bite handler				
C	Dog resource guards/growls over, clasps, etc. stuffed dog				

What are the implications of high and low response scores?

Dogs that show a low threshold for aggression in any category are not only more likely to show aggressive behaviors in the home, they are also more likely to display other severely problematic behaviors. Dogs with any of these issues will require a high level of training on the part of the adopter, and an increased knowledge and desire to learn about body language, canine communication and behavior. Dogs with these issues will almost certainly require management, if not micromanagement, in certain situations, most likely when out in public, quite possibly for the remaining lifetime of the dog. Dogs with these issues are most likely to require lifestyle limitations and accommodations—such as, and depending on the type of low threshold/problematic profile.

For dogs with dog-dog directed reactivity or aggression:

- ❏ Limited places to be walked or exercised, as there are fewer and fewer places to take a dog where there is no risk of encountering either owners with leashed dogs who let their dogs approach and greet, or off-leash and out-of-control dogs that can and will get too close. Often unofficially called The Midnight Walkers Club, owners with dog-dog problematic dogs try to find times where the risk of encountering other dogs is lowest.

- ❏ Adopters of medium- and large-sized dogs in particular will find it challenging and in some cases impossible to sufficiently exercise these dogs.

- ❏ Hiking and being out in nature is often not an option, since the risk of encountering other dogs on most trails today is very high.

- ❏ In many areas and more and more commonly, the only legal, off-leash place to exercise a dog is the public dog park—and these dogs cannot participate, much to the dismay and disappointment of most owners.

- ❏ Walking a dog with dog-dog aggression in any area where the potential to meet an off-leash dog exists (most hiking trails) is irresponsible and dangerous.

Chapter 6

The Additional Tests—Step by Step

Outline of additional tests

1. Teeth Exam

2. Baby Doll Test

3. Toddler Doll Test

4. Cat Test

5. Stranger Tests

    a. Stranger Approachs

    b. Stranger Leaves

The Teeth Exam

The Teeth Exam tests for how quickly the dog reaches an aggression threshold when irritated or frustrated by being *made* to do something he doesn't want to do, or frustrated by being *prevented* from avoiding what he doesn't want to do. If this test seems like we are irritating the dog, *we are*. Indeed, that is the very point.

To assess how the dog might respond in a home with a Level One owner—inexperienced and hence somewhat tentative about handling and communication—it is important to test the dog as if the tester were a Level One owner, with a very light and inexperienced touch, abandoning any handling attempts in which the dog resists or moves in any way. The goal is not to actually examine the dog's teeth! The goal is to get an idea of how much he resists something that he does not want (but is not painful or scary) and in that resistance, when he gets irritated, how quickly he hits his aggression threshold.

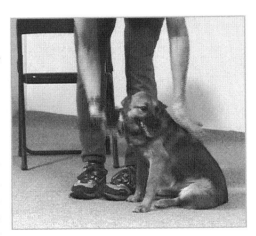

Use a very light and inexperienced touch, abandoning any handling attempts in which the dog resists or moves in any way.

What does the Teeth Exam reveal?

The Teeth Exam reveals what the dog will do when his tolerance level is surpassed and is critical to the safety and success of a pet dog. Aggression during handling, or unwanted or unpleasant interactions, most often exhibited toward familiar people/family members, is a difficult threshold to determine in a shelter dog in a kennel environment. Most shelter dogs are rarely made to do anything they don't want to do, except maybe for being put back in the kennel or during the initial medical exam. Mimicking likely home scenarios in which this type of aggression threshold is reached is impractical. Even the most aggressive dogs rarely show aggression at each and every trigger.

It was necessary, therefore, to develop some form of handling exercise that could irritate a dog, but not cause undue stress or pain or threaten the dog in any way. Also, the procedure needed to have a very low likelihood of triggering a response from a previous traumatic event, one that might push the safe, appropriate pet dog into a freakish or defensive response.

In deciding which part of a dog's body to handle, I considered feet, ears and tail, and nixed them all. I came upon the Teeth Exam, figuring that very few dogs would have come into the shelter with a prior bad experience connected to having their mouths handled. Indeed, I have only two instances where I had to test dogs with a known history of trauma to the mouth. In both cases the dogs passed their Teeth Exams and were successfully adopted.

Safety notes and tips

It can be very dangerous to do this exam on a dog that scored 6 or lower in the Sociability tests. It can be even more dangerous and unwise to do this exam on a dog that froze during the three strokes portion of the Sociability tests.

There is no good way to keep the tester safe during this test, except to limit which dogs to proceed with, and also watch extremely closely for early warning signs—stiffening, dog not moving his feet much, muscling up, freezing, etc. Of course, if this part of the test is skipped due to safety concerns the dog should not be made available as an adoption candidate.

Teeth Exam test step by step

1. Orient yourself so that the dog is at your side, facing the same direction you are.

2. If you are right-handed, have the dog on your left side; if you are left-handed, have the dog on your right side.

3. Gather the leash so that it is almost completely gathered and place it in your dominant hand.

4. Reach with the hand that has the gathered leash for the dog's chin. Keep your palm as flat as possible as you are not trying to "hook" the dog, but rather are attempting to gently come under the dog's muzzle and guide his head toward you.

5. As soon as your hand reaches the dog's chin, reach with two fingers and the thumb of your free hand toward the top of the dog's muzzle, just behind his nose. Your fingers should make contact with the dog lightly and delicately, as if you are reaching for a teacup during high tea with the Queen.

6. The hand under the dog's chin will slightly precede the fingers over the dog's muzzle.

7. Keep your body as upright as possible, and make sure you are not placing your face near the dog's face.

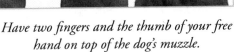

Have two fingers and the thumb of your free hand on top of the dog's muzzle.

8. If and when the dog resists in any way, ducking or pulling away or simply turning his head, let go with both hands (keep holding on to the gathered leash) and try again as shown in the series of five photos below.

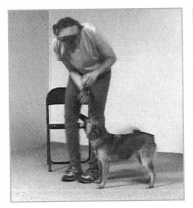
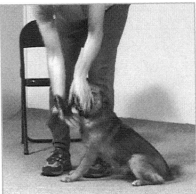
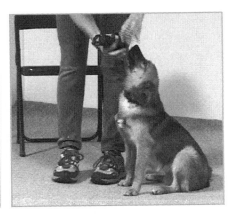
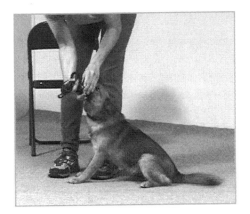
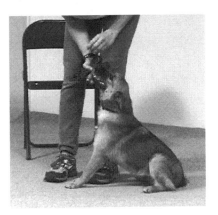

9. You can be talking to the dog in a pleasant and reassuring way.

10. If the dog offers no resistance, and you are able to turn his head toward you, with your dainty fingers pull up lightly on his upper lip to try to expose a canine tooth or any of his front teeth. See if he will allow you to hold and expose a tooth or two for a count of five full seconds.

11. Remember to let go with both hands immediately as soon as he pulls away at all. The goal isn't to actually see his teeth for the five seconds, but rather to see how he responds to your repeated insistence at moving his head and gently trying to part his lips.

12. When you reach for his chin again, try cajoling the dog toward you by tapping your thighs or leaning away.

13. Make 10 attempts.

14. After 10 attempts, if the dog still does not settle or allow any handling, but also does not stiffen, freeze up or snap, the tester can become less hesitant and actually apply slightly more pressure and firmness to the handling and see if the dog defers to this Level Two/ Three handling more readily.

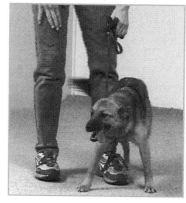

Try cajoling the dog toward you by tapping your thighs.

Notes

☐ Resist the temptation to guide or haul the dog back to your side by using the leash. This type of guidance is how a professional might handle a dog, and not how many inexperienced or hesitant dog owners would do it.

☐ If the dog lies down, rolls or flops, don't pull the dog up with the leash, and don't reach down and do the exam with the dog lying down. Instead, take a step away and cajole the dog enough to get him up, as seen below in the two photos.

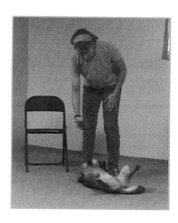 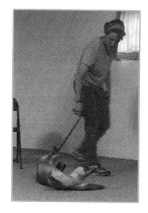

Teeth Exam responses and scoring

Note: All responses are considered more risky with sociability scores of 5 or less.

Note: Score A for adoptable; B for increased risk of aggression; C for high risk of aggression.

Score	Responses	Notes
A	Dog's eyes, head and spine are not aligned, and his body is freely moving	
A	Dog wags tail level, or low and wide	
A	Dog's rear end is wagging along with tail	

Score	Responses	Notes
A	Dog starts with a medium-high tail, but lowers during all repetitions	
A	Dog licks or nuzzles	
A	Dog remains close to tester or moves closer in between repetitions	
A	Dog may paw once or twice, or twist away but accepts all ten attempts, resisting less than 50% of the time	
A	Dog gets progressively more and more excited	
B	Dog re-orients frontally with eyes, head and spine aligned	
B	Dog's arousal level spikes	
B	Dog doesn't move his feet during most of the test and never wags tail or tail is consistently high	
B	Dog uses mouth on tester, even if with no pressure	
B	Dog jumps up and at tester, rebounds off tester's body	
B	Dog's tail is high or raises during exams	
B	Dog makes direct eye contact with tester	
B	Dog head-whips toward tester	
B	Dog head-whips and mouths tester	
C	Dog gets stiff/freezes or remains stiff	
C	Dog growls	

Score	Responses	Notes
C	Dog snarls	
C	Dog snaps	
C	Dog bites or attempts to bite	

Baby Doll test step by step

Preparation

- ❑ The baby doll should be nearby but out of sight. Put a blanket, towel or bedding on the floor next to a chair.

- ❑ The dog should be tethered or on leash. If leashed, have the handle of the leash looped around one of the tester's hands, leaving both hands free to hold the doll.

- ❑ Activate the doll so that it starts making baby sounds. Whoever is handling the baby should treat it exactly as you would a real infant. The tester should do the following:

Step One

1. Pick up the doll and cradle it in your arms.

2. Rock the baby gently and coo to it for a few seconds. If the dog jumps up, exclaim "Ooh, be careful," and snatch the doll protectively up and away and out of reach.

3. Sit in a chair and hold the doll in your lap, facing out toward the dog, so that the baby doll ends up with its eyes staring face to face with the dog. Let the dog investigate. Jostle the doll up and down on your knee.

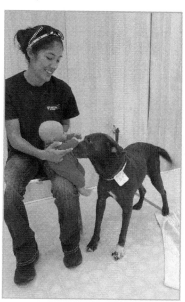 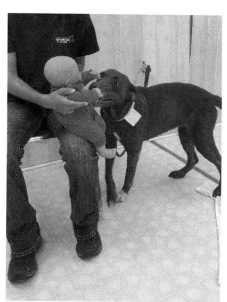 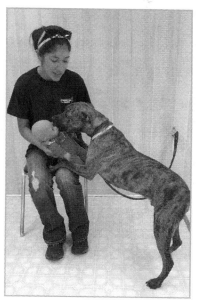

Step Two

1. Place the doll on the floor face up, on top of the blanket or bedding. Allow the dog 15 seconds to investigate the doll.

2. Bend over the doll and pretend to change its diaper, while talking with the dog.

3. Fuss and coo over the doll, giving it all your attention, in baby talk saying things like "How's my little baby? Who's the best baby?" all the while bending all the way down to cuddle the doll.

Baby Doll testing responses and scoring

Note: All responses are considered more risky with sociability scores of 5 or less.

Note: Score A for adoptable; B for increased risk of aggression; C for high risk of aggression.

Score	Responses	Step 1	Step 2	Notes
A	Dog orients toward doll, tail low or level with sweeping or circular wag; head, eyes and spine not aligned			
A	Dog interacts with doll with non-frontal, non-aligned orientation			
A	Dog's eyes are soft and squinty; dog blinks more than once every two seconds			
A	Dog licks or nuzzles doll's fingers or hand gently			
A	Dog is respectful of doll's physical space, tail level or just higher than level (but lower than tail carriage at other environmental arousal)			
A	Dog is indifferent to doll, neither approaches to investigate nor backs off			
B	Dog backs off or avoids doll			
B	Dog steps on doll or engages with rough body contact			

Score	Responses	Step 1	Step 2	Notes
B	Dog approaches doll with frontal body orientation and eyes, head and spine aligned; high tail			
B	Dog's tail remains high, eyes are open wide and hard			
B	Dog raises hackles, either razor thin line between shoulders or full along back			
C	Dog barks at doll			
C	Dog growls at doll			
C	Dog mounts or shoulder swipes doll			
C	Dog arouses suddenly and intensely while orienting toward doll			
C	Dog leaps repeatedly at doll, highly aroused			
C	Dog grabs at doll and shakes			
C	Dog bites at doll			
C	Dog grabs doll by back of neck or head, or grabs the stomach with incisor teeth and picks up doll			

Toddler Doll testing step by step

One person sits or stands with the dog while another handles the doll. The dog will remain on leash.

1. The tester enters the testing area with the toddler doll, grasping its hand as if walking with the child. The toddler doll should be in front of the tester, with its other arm outstretched toward the dog.

2. As the tester and toddler doll approach the dog, the person holding the leash gets up and walks with the dog toward the toddler doll.

3. The tester says to the toddler doll, "Come on, honey, do you want to go say hi to the dog?"

4. The holder asks the tester, "Can my dog say hello to your child?"

5. Allow the dog to interact with the toddler doll. During this time the toddler doll should frontally approach the dog and move into the dog's space and continue to follow and pursue the dog for three seconds.

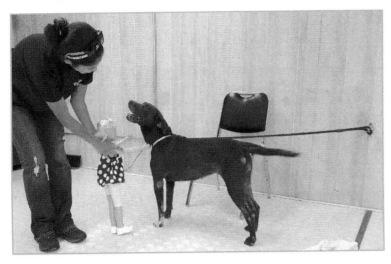 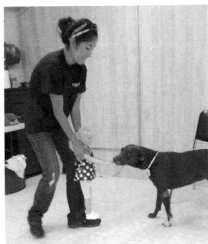

Toddler Doll responses and scoring

Note: All responses are considered more risky with sociability scores of 5 or less.

Note: Score A for adoptable; B for increased risk of aggression; C for high risk of aggression.

Score	Responses	Notes
A	Dog orients toward doll, tail low or level with sweeping or circular wag; head, eyes and spine not aligned	
A	Dog interacts with doll with non-frontal, non-aligned orientation	
A	Dog's eyes are soft and squinty; dog blinks more than once every two seconds	
A	Dog licks or nuzzles doll's fingers or hand gently	
A	Dog is respectful of doll's physical space, tail level or just higher than level (but lower than tail carriage at other environmental arousal)	

Score	Responses	Notes
A	Dog is indifferent to doll, neither approaches to investigate nor backs off	
B	Dog backs off or avoids doll	
B	Dog steps on doll or engages with rough body contact	
B	Dog approaches doll with frontal body orientation and eyes, head and spine aligned, high tail	
B	Dog's tail remains high, dog's eyes are open and wide and hard	
B	Dog barks at doll	
B	Dog growls at doll	
B	Dog raises hackles, either razor thin line between shoulders or full along back	
C	Dog mounts or shoulder swipes doll	
C	Dog arouses suddenly and intensely while orienting toward doll	
C	Dog leaps repeatedly at doll, highly aroused	
C	Dog grabs at doll and shakes	
C	Dog bites or bites at doll	
C	Dog grabs toddler doll by back of neck, hair or head	

The more the child likes dogs, the more potential risk!

While dogs that adore children, seek them out, like to make close, physical contact with them, and show no fear behaviors toward children are often good candidates to live with families or adults likely to have children within the lifetime of the dog, children who adore dogs, and seek them out, and like to hug them and kiss them and interact with them are at much higher risk of getting bitten than are children who ignore, don't care much about, or even who are afraid of and stay away from dogs. The more interaction, the more likely there is to be an aggressive event.

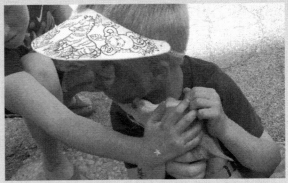

Follow-up observation after testing with dolls

After testing the dog with the baby and toddler dolls, it is important to observe closely any potential adoptive family with the dog. You are observing as much the behavior of the children and parents as you are the dog. There are rowdy, noisy and more interactive (with dogs) children, and there are quieter, more reserved children, or children who are not that interested in dogs. Some dogs thrive on the noise and boisterousness of the household, while others are overwhelmed by this environment and would prefer the quieter household.

Ask different members of the household to call the dog over to them. Ask different members of the family to hug each other or sit close together, or on a lap, and watch the dog's responses. Dogs that strongly orient to one member of the family, particularly an adult member, may have a potential for resource guarding that member from others, particularly from the child(ren). If the dog cuts between the family members or cuts one off from another, this behavior can indicate resource guarding of one family member from another, and children are at particular risk of being bitten. The most successful family dogs are those that seem to give equal attention to all the members.

Adoption guidelines into homes with children

All adoptions into a home with children or visiting children should be done with adequate counseling, educational hand-outs, written behavior and training information for proper supervision, early warning signs of problems and verbal acknowledgment that despite the best, most thorough assessments, we cannot fully predict how a particular shelter dog will behave in the home with real children. Parents, grandparents, aunts, uncles and any adults should proceed with the assumption that the interactions the shelter dog has with children could go wrong or badly, and not the other way around.

Adopters should be made aware that dogs adopted from shelters in the United States have killed adults and children alike, and that children are at greatest risk of injury and disfigurement.

Especially with today's population of shelter dogs—more guarding and fighting dog breed types, more muscular and athletic breed types capable of great harm if there is going to be an incident—placing dogs into environments with children will require from adults, especially in the first few weeks and months, very careful supervision, management and objective observations of behavior.

Cat Test

Cats that flee are more likely to have dogs react badly to them than cats that take a stand and hold their ground with dogs. The Cat Test has limitations in predicting how a dog will respond to a cat that flees, since that is the one thing we cannot really replicate with a fake cat, and it is not fair to torment a real, live cat in the name of testing dogs. Therefore in most cases I recommend using a fake cat. But this test has merit in flushing out the dogs on either temperament/behavior extreme: the dogs that are immediately triggered into a dangerous predatory state at the sight of a cat, or dogs that are so acclimated to cats that they immediately recognize the cat for what it is and offer soft, familiar-with, comfortable-with, sociable responses.

Many shelters have a resident cat (or two, or three…) and often use those cats informally in testing dogs. While that is helpful information to gather about a dog, caution should always be taken when handling/walking dogs past any live creature. It is not safe to assume that a cat can take care of himself around a dog. Or rather, a cat will be able to take care of himself around dogs until one day *he cannot.* No cat should be stressed, tormented or put in danger in order to assess how a dog might respond. However, it is no more humane to send into a home with a cat an unevaluated or inadequately evaluated dog. Dogs with any risky responses are likely to require moderate to high levels of training and intervention on the part of the owner to share a home with a cat.

> ## Be extra cautious placing dogs with cats
> All dog adoptions into a home with a cat should be done with adequate counseling, educational hand-outs, written behavior and training information for proper introductions, warning signs that indicate predatory problems, and safety when the animals are left alone. Especially with today's population of shelter dogs—more guarding/fighting breed types, more dogs with higher prey drive, more large, muscular and athletic dog—placing dogs into homes with cats will require from an owner, especially in the first few weeks/months, vigilance, careful observation and strict management. There is less room for error, and often a first event can be a fatal event. Cats should have free access to many high perches/hiding places, and dog should not be left alone with any cat until the owner is confident the dog is not interested in the cat.

Step One

1. Hold the dog on a leash with about 4 feet of slack.

2. The helper carries the fake cat within visual range of the dog, but well out of leash range.

3. The tester will activate/turn on the cat, place it near the center of the room, facing the dog, and leave the area.

4. The holder should restrain the dog by the leash. Observe the dog's interactions for 30 seconds.

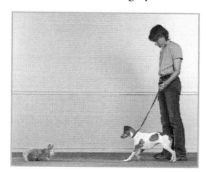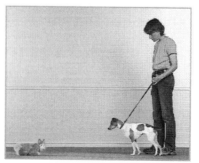

Watch the dog's body language carefully as he approaches and interacts with the cat.

Step Two

Allow the dog to approach the cat and interact with the cat for 20 seconds. If the dog is going to destroy the cat, do not allow access!

Cat test responses and scoring

Note: All responses are considered more risky with sociability scores of 5 or less.

Note: Score A for adoptable; B for increased risk of aggression; C for high risk of aggression.

Scores	Responses	Step 1	Step 2	Notes
A	Dog looks at cat, then disengages on his own to look at tester more than twice while on leash; no tension on leash			
A	Dog sniffs air/cat briefly and disengages from cat within three seconds; no tension on leash			
A	Dog looks at cat, perks up/forward, but relaxes back or disengages within three seconds of visual contact			
A	Dog maintains low level of arousal during entire Cat Test			
A	Dog is uninterested			
A	Dog backs off or avoids cat			
B	Dog bows or barks more than once			
B	Dog bows and/or pokes at cat more than once when he is given access to cat			
B	Dog freezes while staring at cat			

Scores	Responses	Step 1	Step 2	Notes
B	Dog orients toward cat with frontal body orientation and eyes, head and spine aligned, and lowers head/stalks			
B	Dog fixates immediately on cat, with or without trembling or whining, no disconnect within five seconds			
B	Dog arouses suddenly and intensely while orienting toward cat			
C	Dog leaps/lunges repeatedly at cat, highly aroused			
C	Dog grabs at cat and shakes, and you have to buy a new cat			

More than just cats

There is far more to the dog who has killed a cat than simply "finding him a home without a cat." Cat killers generally have a level of predation that far exceeds the level of successful pet. Dogs with that high a level of predation tend to be very difficult to walk or hike with, as they are dangerous and unreliable around livestock and game.

Stranger Tests

The **Stranger Approaches** and the **Stranger Leaves** tests look at the dog's initial responses, and then to the sociable recovery—again, sociability helping to stave off potential aggression problems.

These tests are only for dogs 4 months of age and older. Dogs 4 months and under are too impressionable, in a critical period of development. A potentially scary encounter with a stranger can have a much more profound and lasting effect than the same experience for an older dog. The information gained (e.g., that the dog may be afraid of men, or growl at strangers making eye contact, etc.) is not worth the risk taken. Impressionable puppies have had fewer positive encounters with strangers, and therefore one scary encounter can become more influential, important and detrimental to the puppy than any useful temperament information gleaned from the assessment.

This test further evaluates (along with Cage Presentation) the dog's responses to meeting, greeting and being approached by strangers and unfamiliar people, and having unfamiliar people visit/enter the home. In a home, when a guest knocks at the front door, most dogs will bark for a bit, and then, either with the owner's intervention or on their own, will stop barking and greet the guest in a friendly manner. This is not even just acceptable, but almost ubiquitous. When assessing dogs in a shelter, responses from safe adoption candidates should be quite different, and much less reactive/overt. This is because dogs in shelters are not rooted in or established in the home. They have not laid claim to the territory or resources, and in general are not yet organized and focused in their behaviors, as they would be in a home.

> ## Indoor dogs
> Dogs that have lived indoors will often respond to a knocking with an alert response; dogs that have lived in the back yard and were not part of the indoor household do not usually alert at a knocking.

The Stranger tests are done at the end of the test, when the tester and the dog are more comfortable with each other and the dog more settled into the environment/territory. The stranger knocks at the door, the tester invites him or her in using a slightly nervous voice. The stranger will make no threats, but also no overt social gestures. After the approach the stranger will, still from a distance, try to "make friends" with the dog, by offering lowered, sideways body language, sweet talk, and cajoling.

If there is no one to help who is truly a stranger to the dog, the helper can don a hat or coat, or raise a hood as a disguise.

Stranger Approaches test step by step

Step One (tester's role):

1. Tester sits in a chair with the dog on a short leash, facing wherever the stranger will enter the room.

2. Tester waits until the stranger knocks on the door, then calls out nervously, "Who's there? Come in."

3. As stranger approaches, tester can stroke the dog gently and slowly and offer the type of communication common to many owners: "It's okay, it's okay."

> ## Safety tips for tester
> □ Tester will stop stroking the dog if it distracts the dog.
>
> □ Tester maintains a short leash and a firm grasp of the leash.
>
> □ Tester will not allow the dog to move closer to the stranger at any time.

Step One (stranger/helper's role):

1. Stranger knocks on the door or, if there is no door, will knock on a wall just for the sound effect.

2. Stranger waits for tester to say, "Come in."

3. Stranger enters within visual range and stands upright, eyes, head and spine aligned, arms at side, neutral expression, frontally facing the dog.

4. If dog looks at stranger, stranger will make direct but neutral eye contact with dog for five seconds.

5. If dog doesn't look at stranger, stranger can clear throat to try to catch dog's attention.

6. Stranger will remain for a count of five, even if dog never looks at him/her.

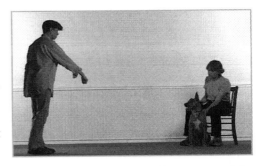

If the dog seems to tolerate the presence of the stranger, he should lean forward toward the dog and hold out his fist with the back of the hand facing upward.

7.   Stranger then bends upper body slightly forward, no more than 10 degrees, holds out a fist with the back of the hand facing upward.

8.   Stranger continues looking at dog and takes two small, very slow steps toward the dog.

9.   Stranger then stops and remains for a count of two.

10. Stranger turns sideways, crouches down and leans away from dog slightly, and smiles and cajoles the dog toward him/her, and attempts to initiate sociability.

Stranger Leaves test

The **tester** keeps a firm hold of a short leash. The **stranger**, abruptly and suddenly, stands up from a crouching position, turns away and rushes toward an exit/door away from the dog.

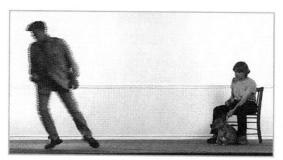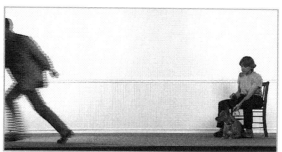

Stranger test responses and scoring

Note: All responses are considered more risky with sociability scores of 5 or less.

Note: Score A for adoptable; B for increased risk of aggression; C for high risk of aggression.

Score	Responses	SA Test	SL Test	Notes
A	Dog wags low and wide, body moves with wagging, with or without attempts to approach stranger			
A	Dog's eyes are squinty and forehead smooth; ears sideways or back			
A	Dog grovels, squints and low wags, with or without attempts to approach stranger			
A	Dog's tail is level or low			

Score	Responses	SA Test	SL Test	Notes
A	Dog is bouncy, distracted, never locks onto stranger, may pounce or bow, doesn't focus on one person or object or in one direction for more than one full second			
A	Dog bows or barks more than once			
A	Dog may stare or sniff air initially, and then disengages on his own			
B	Dog stares at stranger for three full seconds before disengaging on own			
B	Dog takes a shoulder stance, either standing or sitting during any part of the Stranger test, and watches stranger for more than three seconds			
B	Dog may growl briefly and/or back up a step or two			
B	Dog backs away; may or may not try to hide			
B	Dog arouses, pulls and strains toward stranger but scored 5 or fewer sociability points			
B	Dog doesn't move feet at all, or only one or two steps during entire test; body stiff and tense			
C	Dog erupts in barking, no recovery within five seconds			

Score	Responses	SA Test	SL Test	Notes
C	Dog growls and/or snarls, no recovery within five seconds			
C	Dog stiffens, stares, no recovery within five seconds			
C	Dog remains in front of tester, frontal and aligned to stranger for more than five seconds			
C	Regardless of sociability score, dog strains, lunges, arousal spikes, high tail, no recovery within five seconds			

Comments on Stranger Tests

Until a dog reaches maturity, at about 3 to 4 years of age, any fearful or aggressive responses to strangers are still considered progressing or developing. At maturity, responses tend to level off. Therefore, responses seen here in dogs under the age of 2 in general are more worrisome than in mature dogs, since younger dogs still have much potential to get worse.

Dogs that have issues with strangers will need considerably more management, attention to behavior/body language, attention to the environment and situation than dogs without issues with strangers. These include dogs that "don't like/are afraid of men," or are generally suspicious of strangers. More successful placements include owners without the distraction or time-consumption of children. Even homes with older children can be problematic for dogs with stranger issues as pre-teens and teens are often home alone with the dog without adult supervision, and are less likely to perform any management of stranger encounters. Teenagers' friends are often dressed in more intimidating fashion: heavy makeup, multiple piercings, and can be more varied and therefore more intimidating or frightening than regular adult strangers. It is most difficult to control the behavior of other humans, and with stranger issues, successful management and training requires crafting the behavior of every approaching or visiting human as well.

Placing dogs with issues with strangers requires finding a Level Three person or professional dog trainer. Management for a dog with stranger problems is almost always a lifetime endeavor.

CHAPTER 7

Assessing Aggression Thresholds in Owned or Fostered Dogs For Trainers and Behaviorists

Note. Portions of this chapter were first published in *The Chronicle of the Dog,* Association of Professional Dog Trainers.

There are situations in which a dog needs to be assessed, but the dog does not reside in a shelter or kennel environment. There are ways to use portions of the AAP tests and also ways to modify the tests for use in the home, foster-home setting or with an owner present. The following chapters are specifically directed toward:

- ❏ Professional dog trainers and behavior counselors looking to employ portions of the test during their private consultations. This can be very useful when called upon to work with a potentially aggressive or dangerous dog.

- ❏ Rescue or shelter professionals looking to employ portions of AAP on a dog during a surrender interview.

- ❏ Rescue professionals needing to evaluate a dog that is residing in a foster home.

The following modifications can be used in any situation where further behavior information is desired but either the owner is present or the dog is in a home environment. Owned dogs are not all equalized by a shelter or kennel environment, and these dogs already have owners with whom they are, in some form or another, bonded. This can make a difference, as the dog is already attached to someone; he is not, like most shelter dogs, unbonded, detached, seeking a new attachment. So the assessment has to adjust itself, as do some of the responses expected. When interacting with the owned dog, the assessor is, initially, essentially a stranger, and often will remain so during much of the test, whereas in the shelter environment, the assessor is the stranger only during Cage Presentation, and thereafter the shelter dog, looking to form an attachment, starts to bond and consider the assessor as an owner—his safety net.

If you simply walked up to a dog and his owner and started conducting AAP, I would consider this an intrusion, an invasion, and would expect a dog to behave quite differently than if the dog had been in a shelter environment and had lost his attachment to a previous owner. You would not necessarily expect a dog to have the same aggression thresholds with a stranger or unfamiliar person that he would with his owner: If the pizza delivery person arrives at your front door, I wouldn't want to see how quickly your dog hits his aggression threshold when the pizza person places the pizza on the dining room table and reaches down to check your dog's teeth, or does anything to your dog that might be repetitive and irritating. In situations that include stranger or interactions with unfamiliar people, I have a certain expectation that the owner/guardian of the dog is there to protect the dog, as much as possible, from any intrusive, inappropriate or intimidating interactions. The relationship between a stranger and a dog is different than the relationship between an owner and his/her own dog. Therefore the testing has to accommodate this relationship shift.

Paradox of the breed rescuer

Most people who volunteer their time to rescue individuals of their preferred breed are by definition highly experienced people, not just familiar with that breed, but true experts in the breed. When they take a dog into their homes, their communication, handling and savvy with dogs cannot help but come through, which can give them a false sense of the nature of the dog.

Real pet owners with real lives usually behave quite differently than do experienced fosterers and rescuers. Fosterers and rescuers also tend to house multiple dogs at a time, having in the home not just their foster dogs, but their own pet dogs as well, thereby dividing the time spent with each dog into much smaller intervals than would the average owner, who often only has one dog. Real pet owners with only one dog will end up spending much more time, and much more intimate time, with a dog than will most rescuers and fosterers, thereby multiplying the number of interactions and potential for problematic events, which may remain hidden and unknown to the rescuer or fosterer, unless a formal assessment can be done.

During the foster period, a particular dog will live with and be handled by this foster volunteer, expertly, efficiently, and with undesirable behaviors cut off so early in the sequences that the fosterer doesn't even realize they were heading off a problem. This is why so many breed rescue foster homes can house a foster dog for months and witness no aggression, but within two weeks of placing the dog in a home with Level One people, the dog has a bite event. It's easy to blame the Level One adopters for "doing something to the dog" to make him aggressive, but the value of assessing a dog objectively before influencing the dog's behaviors is that it can give a much more accurate picture of how the dog really is and what type of home best suits him. The better a handler or trainer the rescue or foster person is, the less likely they are to notice the dog's actual aggression thresholds. This highlights the need for a formal assessment!

Words of caution for trainers and behavior professionals

In my experience it can be very difficult, if not near impossible, for a good trainer to *not train a dog!* What I mean by this is that it seems very difficult for a trainer to simply assess and observe a dog and not want to immediately start training or modifying the dog's behavior. While this is useful during any training or behavior modification consult, it will interfere with a proper assessment. If you decide to assess a dog, then you must withhold your desire to influence behavior/train the dog! Mixing the two will give you an unclear and potentially dangerously false assessment.

It is perfectly okay to make a decision not to assess a dog and to instead start training or modifying behavior, but once you interrupt the assessment and start shaping, modifying or cutting off behaviors, the assessment becomes invalid.

As a dog trainer and behavior consultant, it is possible to be a successful practitioner without a thorough knowledge of temperament. But understanding temperament and being able to read a dog's basic personality traits and aggression thresholds can greatly enhance a trainer's ability to make a diagnosis and design a much more customized training and behavior modification plan. It can also keep the trainer safer. By learning to assess a dog, and by performing or observing hours and hours of assessments, you can start to "thin slice" dog behavior—find patterns or make decisions from minimal amounts of information.

The most important components of the test for the in-home evaluator are the tests assessing a dog's responses:

- ❑ To house guests, meter readers, delivery people and/or approaching visitors using the Stranger tests.
- ❑ During handling, and to being made to do something he doesn't want to do, or prevented from doing something he *does* want to do, often frustration-based aggression using, for example, the Teeth Exam, with the owners performing the tests.

❑ Around resources such as a cloth or squeak toy, a pig's ear and the dog's food bowl using the Resource Guarding test.

❑ Around public or unfamiliar dogs while on leash using the Dog-Dog test.

❑ Observing sociability toward each owner and toward the assessors using the Sociability test.

With an in-home visit, as compared to a shelter dog evaluation, you can, through careful mining and excavation, obtain a lot of realistic and useful behavior history and temperament information. With a shelter dog, you usually don't have an owner to ask, and even when you do have the surrenderer present, good information can be challenging to obtain due to time constraints, owner bias, guilt and protectiveness over the dog's behaviors because of the fear of euthanasia. I am in no way saying owners are pathological liars or are deliberately withholding the truth. In fact, a study done in 1998 by Patronek, DiGiacomo, and others of Tuft's University School of Animals and Public Policy, interviewed people surrendering their dogs and cats to two different shelters in the Midwest. It showed that in all cases, owners were most worried that their pet might be euthanized, and spent an average of eight months deliberating over whether to surrender or keep their pet. Most importantly, the number one reason for surrender was behavior problems. So the owner bias is toward presenting their pet in the very best light, with the fear that their pet might be euthanized. Also, pet owners are not professionals, and do not organize, categorize or understand behavior and aggression thresholds the same way professionals do, so when asked one-line questions on reasons for surrender, they will give one-line answers that will not accurately represent the behavior/temperament of their pet.

Often a dog's behavior history shows a fairly limited and fairly inhibited bite history, but the presenting dog is, to put it rather unscientifically, *scary*. Sometimes dangerous dogs, the ones that are really aggressive, have aggressive events *infrequently*. In my experience, their aggression levels are so high they rarely feel enough conflict to escalate into aggression. A temperament test can help you determine the future risk—the dog's aggression thresholds. There should be no need to wait for a real live violent event to predict violence.

Getting solid and useful behavior information from an owner hinges more on *how* the interview is conducted than on *what* the actual interview questions are.

Modifying AAP for use in private settings

Modifying the AAP for use in the private setting will include instructing the owner to perform some of the procedures. This is to help determine the dog's responses to his actual owner. In the shelter setting, we are trying to determine how the dog would ultimately respond to a future owner, and what level of skill and experience that future owner should have if adopting that particular dog. In the private setting, we *have* the owner, and want to determine his or her level of skill and confidence. What you do will depend on a number of variables reviewed below.

Levels of dogs, levels of owners

Remember that AAP divides dogs into three "levels" or categories:

1. **Level One** dogs are the easiest, most compliant, friendliest and gentlest of dogs. They are often successful in families with young children (under 7 years old), or with people inexperienced and unfamiliar with dogs. These Level One dogs are all but extinct.

2. **Level Two** dogs are compliant and friendly, but may be a little smarter, more pushy, and more creative than Level One dogs. They may also be more appropriate for children 8 years and older. Level Two dogs have, like Level One dogs, high aggression thresholds in all categories, and are at low risk for highly problematic behavior and/or aggressive events.

3. **Level Three** dogs are dogs that also have high aggression thresholds in all but maybe one category, so may be slightly more difficult in the real world than the Level Ones and Twos. Level Three dogs may like to initiate things or be pushy. They are dogs that would do best with a working outlet (i.e., agility, scent work, hiking, Frisbee, flyball, etc.) to truly be satisfied and successful. Level Three dogs may be bold and fearless, or anxious, nervous, fearful types, but they are dogs that will likely require some knowledge of behavior/body language, and would do best with more extensive training and management.

These three levels represent dogs that are *unlikely* to be a menace to society, or cause any harm. These are dogs, for better or worse, that you would not mind having as next door neighbors; that you wouldn't mind adopting out to your 8-year-old daughter's piano teacher; these are dogs with medium to high aggression thresholds, that are not going to cause an event that requires medical attention. With Level One, Two and Three dogs, even if your clients and owners are unable to comply with your behavior modification plans, or they were truly incompetent and unlikely to learn the skills you are recommending for training and management, the likelihood of a hospitalizing event or worse is extremely low.

Dogs with lower thresholds for aggression make more problematic pets overall, even if the primary complaint from the owner is not aggression. Dogs with little to no sociability, low aggression thresholds, and often a teeny bit of fear mixed in are dogs that pose the greatest risk for harm.

AAP also divides humans into three "levels" or categories of ownership:

1. **Level One** people are inexperienced people with children aged 7 and under already in the home, young children "on the way," and/or young children in the environment—such as grandchildren, nieces and nephews, or they live in an apartment building with children riding with them in elevators and all around the property. They often lead busy lives and dogs are not (yet?) first and foremost on their minds and in their plans. Level One owners have no "feel" for dogs, literally aren't used to petting, holding a leash, grooming, and all the various tiny parts that come with living with a dog.

2. **Level Two** people may be equally inexperienced or may be experienced but have no children, or children 8 years and older. Level Two owners also include anyone with confidence and clear body language skills: "leader-type" people who like to learn about behavior and body language and are naturally clear communicators, never hesitant in their handling and could likely handle a slightly more challenging dog. Level Two adopters may also be people who are planning to make the dog a more central part of their lives than Level One adopters (often childless or empty nesters who will make the dog the focus of their lives).

3. **Level Three** people are professionals, either trainers, sports hobbyists (Nosework, agility or flyball folks, etc.) or volunteers or staff at a shelter willing to live with a challenging dog that requires some kind of management for life. Many people are Level One or Two humans about to be inspired, either by a difficult/challenging dog, or by such an amazing dog that they will try out a dog sport, attend a dog camp with their dog, attend a lecture, read a couple of books and voila! They become a Level Three professional!

When assessing an owned dog, one of the goals is to try to figure out what "level" owner(s) the dog has lived with, and whether or not the combination has been successful. Some surrenders happen because of financial or life crises, and are not the fault of the dog or the match between dog and human(s). Other surrenders are due to a mismatch or due to the temperament and behavior of the dog, but are described with one-line answers to the one-line question of "Why can't you keep this dog?":

- ❑ "The dog got too big."
- ❑ "We don't have enough time."
- ❑ "The dog needs more room to run."

And many more. AAP can transcend judgments and criticism of the surrenderer into objective knowledge of the dog's basic temperament, his best possible future people and home, if he tests out as safe enough.

When to use AAP during a training or behavior consultation

I will use portions of AAP during a consult for a variety of reasons, but I do not routinely test a dog's temperament during a consult. Understand that each time a dog shows an aggressive response during any part of the test, he is practicing that aggression and getting incrementally worse. This is an undesirable but necessary consequence in any testing of a shelter dog, which is an unknown. As a private trainer/behavior counselor, the decision must be made whether the risk of making the dog's behavior slightly worse will be worth the knowledge gained.

I will use the test in these circumstances:

1. To get a read on the dog's capabilities and thresholds for aggression when I am uncertain just how far the dog could or would go in a given situation.

2. When the dog is owned by a couple instead of single person, and clearly one partner gets a very different response from the dog while the other partner is in a little disbelief; or if one partner is clearly afraid of the dog and the other partner is not, and I need that issue flushed out and the problem illustrated to the clients, instead of having me point out the issue.

3. When the dog is new to the family and they want an evaluation done.

4. When the clients are worried about the dog's behavior and are expecting a baby.

5. When a client seems in complete denial of the severity of the dog's problem; there are times as a trainer that you need to shock the owners into acknowledging just how aggressive the dog is to convince one or both owners of the danger they are in, or the risk to their child(ren).

I will *not* use the test:

1. When doing so would cause the dog to practice an aggressive response to a trigger that has already been worked with, and with ample progress.

2. When the clients are hiring me for one particular behavior issue and I see another issue in the dog, but the owners don't find this other issue a problem and testing the dog could aggravate or bring to life that other issue.

3. If it is not possible to keep the owners or myself safe during testing.

Observation: Being good at reading temperament means being able to read subtle body language

When people hear about assessments, particularly shelter dog assessments, they may think that it doesn't apply to them, or that because they don't work in a shelter, they don't have to learn or know about assessments. What makes me want to leap on top of a mountain and scream out to all the dog people out there is, "Assessments are about LEARNING TO READ A DOG!!!" Assessments exist so that after maybe 100 or 1,000 dogs, you can simply thin-slice and look at a dog and *in an instant,* know his aggression thresholds and predict his behaviors. What dog lover would not want this skill?

By understanding temperament and increasing your powers of observation of body language and communication between owner and dog, you can gain a much-expanded view of the dog and the home situation. Trainers can then create a much more successful training or behavior modification plan, as well as determine how safe the situation is or isn't. Risk assessment for aggression is much better determined with an understanding of temperament, and trainers can make a safer prognosis and better determine emotional, physical and financial liability.

Assessing sociability in the home

Probably the most important part of AAP is the *sociability* of the dog. When shelter dogs come out of their cage for testing, it is more likely that the pet or companion dogs (as opposed to fighting or guarding dogs) will come out and seek companionship from a human. In other words, they will initiate a sociable interaction with the tester because that is what they missed the most in the kennels.

In my experience, most shelter dogs, after a few days, often un-bond, or un-attach or *detach* from any previous owner. Therefore, when a tester takes a dog out of his cage for an evaluation, the dog is often quite ready to re-bond, to reattach himself to a new person. Most pet dogs will come out of their kennels and offer sociable contact with the tester.

Going into a home with an owned, loved and attended dog, you cannot necessarily expect that dog to immediately initiate social contact with *you.* The owned dog is usually not deprived of human contact. The owned dog has an owner, and therefore you are a stranger. Many dogs don't automatically seek out social contact with a stranger. Some highly sociable dogs do, but owned dogs shouldn't be penalized for not initiating social contact with you early on in the visit.

Dogs with more than one owner

For dogs living with more than one owner, responses that are vastly different for each owner, particularly when dealing with a dog with aggression issues, can indicate a situation that is extremely difficult to resolve successfully, and the dog poses much more of a risk for the family. The risk is greatest for the owner who gets less of a sociable response from the dog. If owners are in this situation, but with the added detail (gathered from a behavior history or a trainer's observation) that one owner uses physical force, physical confrontation or physical punishment to control the dog (when dealing with aggression issues) *and the other owner does not,* also greatly increases the risk to that family and makes even more remote the possibility of a successful outcome. If the same situation exists, with yet one more added detail (gathered from a behavior history or by observation): *one owner is afraid of the dog,* then the prognosis is even more dismal, and the risk to the family is again, hugely increased.

Testing procedures for sociability in the home

It is quite easy to observe the natural interactions between dog and owner as you are taking a behavior history. A good portion of the private consult should allow for the owner to express himself, talk freely about the dog, and choose what characteristics and events to share and in what order. While this is happening, you can observe the interactions.

1. Ask one owner at a time (adults only) to cajole the dog over to him or her, without using treats or toys. The dog should be somewhere other than near the owner when he is cajoled.

2. Then ask one owner at a time to gently-but-firmly pet/stroke the dog from the base of his neck down the back to the base of the tail. Pause. Repeat the stroke. Pause, and repeat a third time.

3. The owner(s) can be sitting down or standing for these tests.

Safety tips

- Before you begin, you will need to talk the owners through this, tell them when and how to stroke and when to pause.

- Remember to ask each owner, before coaching them to do it, if s/he feels comfortable doing this!

- Remember *not* to do this if the dog already has a bite history (owner-directed) and/or either owner is afraid of the dog, or should be, or if the dog looks ready to bite again, and soon.

As an experienced trainer, you don't likely need to use the scoring system that I recommend in a shelter environment; rather you can rate dogs as more or less sociable by focusing on the following factors:

A dog that is more sociable will:

- ❑ Come readily and eagerly, little cajoling is needed
- ❑ Approach unaligned (head, eyes and spine offset)
- ❑ Lower the base of the tail the closer he comes to the tester
- ❑ Smooth out his forehead and put his ears back/sideways
- ❑ Wag his tail low and wide-sweeping
- ❑ Show a cashew/crescent shaped approach

A dog that is less sociable will:

- ❑ Require multiple attempts before approaching
- ❑ Approach with head, eyes and spine aligned
- ❑ Keep his tail high or raise it upon approach
- ❑ Have a stiff body

In a shelter dog assessment, sociability gets scored/quantified by giving the dog one point for every two seconds of sustained gentle physical contact, while orienting toward the tester—excluding mounting, sniffing and biting (any teeth touching human skin or clothes). Even if the observer is unsure of whether the physical contact made by the dog is "gentle" or "brutal," "sociable" or "threatening," the process of counting (one Mississippi, two Mississippi, three Mississippi, etc.) can most often define the intention of the dog: brutal, non-sociable contact rarely lasts a few seconds. The occasional exception of non-sociable contact that gets scored as sociable because the dog is indeed making physical contact lasting two seconds or longer tends to come in the form of intrusive, space-taking approaches, stiff body, or a slow approach, usually climbing onto the lap while the tester is seated, accompanied by a tensing of the muscles.

In the home assessment for sociability, there is less quantifying and more gathering of subtle body language to fill in your overall picture of the relationship between dog and family.

During sociability observations, there are a number of behaviors to be observed and noted. There are also small red flag behaviors and threat displays that should be observed.

Red flag behaviors

Red flag behaviors are those that, alone, don't indicate much of a potential for aggression, but when combined with other red flag behaviors, or in multiples, can indicate greater potential for aggression. Therefore, each individual red flag behavior should be noted—as inconsequential or as insignificant as it may seem. At the end of the evaluation, it is the accumulation—or lack of—red flag behaviors that help create an overall risk assessment.

Even red flag behaviors with possible "excuses" for existing (e.g., the dog "shakes off" because maybe he has an ear infection, or the dog rubbed his shoulder against his owner because he was itchy, etc.) should still be noted, and additional notes can be made if the evaluator believes there is a "reason" for the behavior excusing the dog from risk. This is to keep the assessment objective and less emotional.

In observing dogs, attention to behavioral detail is critical. While each individual behavior may seem insignificant or explicable, a combination or accumulation of such behaviors could indicate a more risky dog, with more potential for violence. Our job as trainers and behavior counselors is to help predict and thwart future problematic or violent events.

The following red flag behaviors are important to be aware of:

1. **Anal swipe.** This is when the dog's anus makes swiping contact with the owner(s) or you (often as the dog turns around while keeping his tail high) or with furniture or walls in the area.*

2. **Anus touch.** This is when the dog actually rests his anus on a human or on furniture. Often the dog will back up, keeping his tail high, and plant his anus on the person. The most common way for the anus to touch is when the dog sits on the person's shoe.*

3. **Shake off.** This is when the dog starts with his head/neck and moves quickly in a twisting motion that travels down the dog's body ending with his tail. Red flag if noted after contact with a person.

4. **Shoulder rub.** This is when the dog makes contact with a person or furniture by first touching with the back of his neck/shoulder area, and smearing/rubbing/swiping the rest of his body across the person or furniture. This looks similar to when the dog rolls on a smelly item in the backyard, except the dog is upright.*

5. **Frontal orientation during interaction.** This is when the dog squares off to the person when making eye contact or interacting with a person in any way. In the competition obedience ring, the position would constitute a near-perfect score for a "front." The dog may be sitting or standing.

6. **Head, eyes, spine aligned.** This is when the dog aligns his eyes, head and spine while interacting with a person. Sometimes this alignment can occur even as the dog passes in front of the plane of the person.

7. **Chin high.** This is when the dog keeps his chin high, his head and shoulders erect and hence his throat exposed. It may be a subtle form of space-taking.

8. **Too-wide panting.** This is when the dog pants in situations that temperature-wise or activity-wise don't call for panting, and the dog's mouth is often wider than necessary. The tongue may protrude beyond the dog's lower jaw. The rate of respiration during this panting is not much faster than normal breathing. Dogs that pant "too wide" often keep their chins high as well.

9. **Tail high or raises higher.** Watch the base of the dog's tail, as during arousal or curiosity the dog's tail will be carried at a certain level. When interacting with a person the dog may keep his tail level or actually raise it higher than during arousal or curiosity. Red flag interactions are when the dog doesn't lower or worse, raises his tail when interacting with people.

10. **Eyes wide and round (hard eyes).** This is when the dog keeps his eyes wide and round, the pupil is often reflective, and this is called a "hard eye." The brow may be furrowed.

11. **Blinking less than once every two seconds.** Make sure to count full seconds (one Mississippi, two Mississippi, etc.).

*These behaviors group into what I consider scent-marking behaviors.

Threat displays

Threat displays are more potent than red flag behaviors. The following behaviors are threat displays and may warn of actual intent for possible aggression.

1. Freeze

2. Stiffening up, or remaining stiff

3. Muscling up

4. Muzzle bop, tap or punch

5. Mouth on human

6. Teeth on human

7. Growl

8. Snap

Don't be too quick to judge if...
Remember not to judge any untrained or ill-mannered behaviors (jumping up, pawing), or be too quick to start training, as many sociable dogs offer their sociability in untrained or ill-mannered ways!

Recap: assessing sociability

To recap, sociable dogs, when interacting with their owners, generally use the following body language:

❑ Tail carriage will be lower when interacting with the owner than during arousal. The base of the dog's tail is the part to watch. Even in Rottweilers, Australian Shepherds, Corgis, etc. it can be easily observed. Northern breeds, with curled or double curled tails, are also able to relax and lower their tails. Obviously a Pug will not lower his tail like a Whippet, but both have the ability to raise and lower the bases of their tails. The only breed types exempt from this observation should be the corkscrew tails (Boston Terriers, French Bulldogs, English, and some Old English Bulldogs, etc.).

❑ Ears will go back, or remain back, while the dog's forehead will relax and his eyes will squint in response to a smile or sweet-talk from the owner directed to the dog.

❑ Sociable dogs seek attention and interact with their owners without aligning their eyes, heads and spines. One of these three body parts will be out of alignment during most social interactions between dog and owner.

❑ Eye contact from the sociable dog to his owner usually includes blinking more than once every two to three seconds.

Sociable dogs will be equally affectionate whether they initiate the interaction or the owner initiates. In most healthy relationships, the owner initiates and terminates the majority of the interactions.

Beware of the subtle differences between the truly sociable dog and the demanding, attention-seeking dog. The demanding dog often:

❑ Initiates and terminates most of the interactions.

❑ Does not comply when the owner requests a behavior.

❑ Keeps his chin high and throat exposed when interacting with the owner.

❑ Keeps his tail high or even sometimes raises his tail while interacting with the owner.

❑ Is physically intrusive into the owner's personal and physical space, i.e., jumps up *into* the owner and often expels air out of the owner's mouth with the force of his paws; lunges toward the owner's face and causes the owner to back off or put up his hand to protect himself.

❑ Never or seldom softens his eyes. The eyes of the demanding dog are often fully open, wide, and round, and pupils are dilated and reflecting dark-bluish light.

❑ If panting, pants wider than necessary, keeping his tongue mostly inside his mouth, and is more often panting when there seems no need for panting (it's not hot, and the dog hasn't just exercised extensively, etc.).

Some more observations on sociability

Although just sociability was covered in this first section, a lot of important information can be gleaned by the observant dog trainer. I think the more sociable the dog, the bigger the buffer against a lot of aggression issues. In particular, I have seen that high sociability seems to help the dog inhibit his bite, especially in aggression directed toward the owner in the home. The more sociable, the easier I know it will be for owners to implement a training program, since they're starting with a dog that already finds them reinforcing. Non-sociable dogs work for treats and toys, but may not find praise/petting or smiles and attention influential at all. Many sociable dogs find simply being with their owners reinforcing.

Having trained sociable and non-sociable dogs side by side in a variety of different dog sports, it has been my experience that the sociable dogs are more forgiving of any lapses in timing I might have and will continue to work despite late reinforcers, missed markers and my generally sloppy training. This is especially so in the higher levels of training. Non-sociable dogs are less forgiving. A late reinforcer and the dog checks out, and goes off for something more interesting. It is a bit like training a farm animal. This is not to say that any dog that checks out during (or leaves) a training session is likely unsociable, rather that unsociable dogs are more likely to check out and leave.

The more a dog naturally looks at his owners, the easier attention is to capture, reinforce, perpetuate and increase in frequency. That is in no way saying that attention isn't an easy trick to teach. It is, but in the face of a distraction, the sociable dog at the very least finds his owner reinforcing, whereas the unsociable dog may be 100% distracted and the delivery of reinforcers needs to be practically flawless to keep that attention.

In certain higher-level competition training, the opposite can often be true. The least sociable dogs are often a blast to teach easy, new behaviors, especially during the early stages of training (like sit and eye contact, lie down, etc). If food or toy motivated enough, they often offer keen attention during these training sessions, and are not easily interrupted by the need to come over and just get petted or cuddle. They are less sensitive to the moods of their handler. In a higher pressure training/competition session, where the owner is upset, angry or disappointed in either him or herself or the dog, the sociable dog tends to notice and become anxious, while the unsociable dog could not care less, and prefers to just get on with the training.

For dogs with separation problems:

- ❑ This can be extremely restrictive for adopters, as often even just a quick trip to the grocery store can cause the dog to perform whatever distress-related behaviors he comes with.

- ❑ Behavior modification treatment plans are often lengthy, intensive and tedious. Any progress can be sabotaged with one single separation event. These treatment plans are difficult for most adopters to execute successfully.

- ❑ Separation problems can cause constant worry whenever the owner is out of the house, negatively affecting any social outings.

- ❑ There is virtually no home environment where a dog will not have to, at some point, be left alone.

Assessing thresholds for aggression directed toward familiar people in the home

In assessing dogs, one of the most difficult problems to predict can be aggression directed at the owner(s) when the dog is made to do something he doesn't want to do, or is prevented from doing something he wants to do—often associated with frustration. One of the reasons I think this is so difficult to predict is that it often has as much to do with the communication from human to dog as it does from dog to human. We currently have no system for assessing human/adopter behavior. Before the advent of temperament assessments, shelters would adopt out any dog that *seemed* friendly in the kennels. Often the dogs that *seem* the friendliest (dogs that "appear friendly," but do not actually behave in a friendly way) are asocial, assertive dogs that are not showing any overt aggression because they are not being challenged or pushed in any way at the shelter. The shelter/kennel environment is such that a dog is rarely confronted with doing something he doesn't want to do, or restrained from doing what he does want to do, with the exception of going back into his kennel. We frequently see bites that occur during the lunging/barking phase of being walked down the kennel aisles, or walked past another dog outside. In a home environment, with certain types of owners, a dog also may never be made to do something he doesn't want to do, and a sometimes very intricate dance is performed throughout each day as the owner avoids any type of confrontation, consciously and often subconsciously thwarting aggressive events. This is one of the reasons it is so important to assess a dog that is being re-homed—as just taking a behavior history may display a dog with no overt aggressive events, but an assessment will reveal all the latent aggression, the aggression tamped down underneath elaborate rituals that avoid conflict. The next owner will not know any of these rituals or dances, and could experience a much more aggressive dog than did the previous or current owner.

Another big reason for the difficulty in flushing out this type of aggression is the fact that most dogs in shelters are highly aroused, over-stimulated and disorganized. For certain types of aggression in the home, in order to hit threshold, the dog must first organize and focus. This hardly ever occurs at the shelter, but in the home, in a more intimate setting, with fewer distractions, the dog has a calm and focused demeanor, and the organization and focus happen more frequently.

A dog in a shelter is difficult to evaluate for this particular type of aggression for a few reasons. In my experience, much of the risk of this type of aggression depends on the communication with and from the owner(s). And this in itself seems to work in two separate ways. The confident and skilled owner, who sets clear limits and communicates calmly and frequently with the dog, often can establish and maintain an obvious and gentle claim over rules, intentions and resources. The best owners do so without ever having to resort to threat displays, "alpha" manipulations or physical violence. In that situation, the low-threshold dog can often exist without any serious aggressive events. On the other hand, many owners co-exist successfully without any serious aggressive events from the low-threshold dog by remaining completely passive and permissive, and dare I say clueless to the dog's initiatives and communication over rules and resources. So having the owner(s) present to reveal what level of handler the dog has lived with, and what level would be best for his future, can be a gift.

Aggression thresholds are reached when there is a conflict. Whether the owner is above that conflict point, or well below it is almost (*almost*) a moot point. Either way, there may be no overt aggressive event. But when re-homing a dog, particularly an adult dog with mature capabilities for harm, knowing where that threshold lies is supremely important in determining the safety for his future.

Problematic behaviors directed toward people in the home

From my experience, I have seen two main issues in the home from dogs that have low thresholds for aggression in response to handling/frustration/being made to do something they don't want to do:

1. Actual aggression, or near-aggressive events.

2. Extreme or severe problem behaviors other than overt aggression, e.g., problems being left alone, extraordinary destructiveness, huge barking problems, etc.

In a home, aggression often occurs in such situations as:

- ❏ When the owner tries to rouse the dog from a comfortable resting place.
- ❏ When the owner tries to move the dog off his or the owner's bed.
- ❏ When the owner tries to put the dog into a crate, or take him out of a crate.
- ❏ When the owner tries to hold or grab the dog by the collar to prevent the dog from doing something he wants to do.
- ❏ When being handled, groomed, touched, hugged or restrained.

How to modify the Teeth Exam for use in the in-home setting

The beauty of using this portion of AAP in the home, with the owners present, is that the Teeth Exam procedures are done by each adult owner, and you need not instruct anyone on what level to do—*this is where they show you what level they are!* Here is how to proceed:

1. First ask one adult owner to please lift the dog's lips and expose his front teeth by placing one hand underneath the dog's chin and the other hand over the dog's muzzle.

2. If they can hold the lips parted for a count of three that would be great.

3. Whether or not they can be successful for the count of three, I instruct them to attempt, pause, let go, and repeat. I usually have each owner do it three times in a row.

The repetition of the test is important as it shows you the escalation (or lack thereof) of the dog's communication. I then instruct the other adult member of the household (if there is one) to do the same.

I will stop the test at any point if I believe the dog is about to bite, or the person is visibly afraid. I typically do not ask the adults to do this if children under the age of 8 years are present, as I worry that the children will misunderstand and start performing a Teeth Exam on the dog, which could pose a risk. I always first ask if the owner is comfortable performing the task. Then I explain briefly that I am looking for responses from the dog to this exercise, and that it can give me a clearer view of the dog's tolerance to doing things he may not want to do.

I use the Teeth Exam portion of AAP when:

- ❏ I want to gauge each owner's handling abilities with the dog, to see how the dog responds to each adult owner.
- ❏ I want to see if what the owners interpret about the compliance of the dog jives with the dog's actual compliance.

- ❑ I want to see if the dog is living with two very different types of adults—one with great authority, strength and confidence, and the other without.
- ❑ I want to make sure no adult owner is afraid of the dog.
- ❑ I want to know if the owners interpret the ease in making their dog do something he didn't want to do only because I can see via the behavior history or by observation that they've never made the dog do something he does not want to do.

Responses to expect from dogs during the Teeth Exam

Risky responses:
- ❑ Watch for any stiffening, hardening or tightening from the dog.
- ❑ Watch for any freezes, including whether the dog pulls away and freezes, or tucks his chin and freezes—these are all reasons to stop the test and have the owner cease immediately.
- ❑ Watch for the dog that spikes in arousal and begins to charge at or leap repeatedly at the owner, especially with a frontal and aligned body orientation.
- ❑ Watch for the dog that gets "mouthy, " i.e., begins to pant with a very wide jaw, touches his teeth repeatedly to the owners hands or body, clacks his teeth or places his mouth on the owner.

Healthy responses:
- ❑ Any avoidance behaviors that are presented once or twice and then the dog changes tactics—e.g., the dog leaps out of reach, then ducks backwards, then comes closer and offers appeasement gestures (licking, curled spine with ears back, soft eyes, relaxed forehead, low tail wag, etc.).
- ❑ Compliance and relaxation after three or four attempts by the owner.
- ❑ The dog sighs and rests his chin on the tester's hand, frequent blinking (more than once every two seconds) with relaxed forehead.

Communication between dog and owner during the Teeth Exam

Level One owners:
- ❑ Will usually cajole the dog over instead of physically manipulating the dog.
- ❑ Do not usually like to exert more physical strength in handling the dog than the dog exerts upon the owner.
- ❑ Will usually let go of the dog's muzzle if the dog resists or pulls back in any way.
- ❑ Will often take the cues from the dog, as opposed to ignoring the cues from the dog and proceeding on with the task—i.e., if the dog jerks his head away before the allotted time, the owner will let go, if the dog tucks his chin, the Level One owner will accommodate and try to part the dog's lips while the dog's chin is tucked, or if the dog lies down, the owner will get down on the floor and do the Teeth Exam down there.

Level Two owners:
- ❑ Will handle the dog with confidence, without hesitation, and often willingly exert enough physical strength in handling to hold the dog still.
- ❑ Will usually grip the dog's head or body tighter, or will reposition him or herself to get a better hold of the dog if the dog pulls away.

❑ Usually seem to know exactly the places on the dog's body to touch in order to gently and effectively get the job done.

❑ Will persist in the task even if the dog continues to resist.

❑ May get on the floor or roll around with the dog if the dog uses rolling around techniques to thwart the Teeth Exam.

Responses to expect from owners during the Teeth Exam

I've found this test very useful during private consults as well as surrender interviews for many different reasons.

❑ I have been reassured after witnessing an owner or both owners confidently handle a large or giant breed-type dog that is presenting with potentially workable and manageable stranger-aggression issues during the Teeth Exam. This is important in my assessment of overall management possibilities, and whether or not I feel it is at all safe to give these owners a training and behavior plan while out in public. If the owners are intimidated by their large or giant (and size is relative) dog, I hesitate to send them out in public to work with their dog—I think it poses a greater risk to the public.

❑ I've had owners finally admit to being afraid of their dogs, or one owner in a two-owner household will, during the Teeth Exam. This has been critical during consultations regarding safety of the dog after the arrival of a baby or newly adopted child. Owners who are intimidated by their dog (but the owners haven't acknowledged or admitted that to either themselves or their partners) are often in denial about the risk the dog now poses. This is also a critical and honest revelation a couple must have in order to proceed with whatever course of action is necessary, whether or not they have a new baby or child in the household. No one should live in fear of violence from a dog or human.

❑ It has been invaluable during surrender interviews, where the dog has had no history of overt or damaging aggression, but the dog clearly presents as a dangerous, non-re-homeable dog, and you must gently take the owner(s) on a journey to understand that if they surrender their dog to your shelter the dog will likely be euthanized, or that if they try to place the dog privately, that the dog is dangerous. At my shelter, we believe the public has a right to know why we euthanize—for temperament, behavior or loss of quality of life.

❑ The Teeth Exam has been valuable in showing me a large discrepancy in the skills and handling ability between each owner, and a dog that behaves vastly differently with each owner. This is useful because sometimes one owner doesn't witness or believe the dog behaves any differently with the other owner, and won't change his or her behaviors with the dog as per your recommendations, and revealing out in the open how the dog behaves differently, without humiliating or blaming either owner is critical to success. The same holds true for the situation where one owner is heavy-handed and uses physical techniques to intimidate the dog into behaving, and the other owner is soft or more tolerant of the dog, and the dog is suffering in more ways than just behaviorally because of this.

Conclusions regarding the Teeth Exam

For use during private behavior consultations, the Teeth Exam is valuable in identifying serious relationship issues that could hamper or prevent a successful outcome.

For use during surrender interviews, the Teeth Exam holds exceptional value in identifying what level owner the dog has been living with (either successfully or unsuccessfully) and what level owner might work best for this dog in his next home, as well as flushing out the dog's potential for harm/aggression to his next owner. Many dogs have lived successfully with their original owner(s) from puppyhood and have had no aggression events in the original home, but re-homing the same dog *as an adult dog* into a new household poses a much larger risk. Explaining this to the owners of the dog can be difficult without the visible, observable communication that comes out during a Teeth Exam.

Using the Stranger tests in the home

In the shelter setting, the Stranger test is done toward the end of the assessment, to allow the dog to get acclimated and comfortable both in the room and with the tester. In the in-home setting, the evaluator *is* the stranger when he or she arrives. The dog is already quite comfortable in the home and quite bonded with the owner. Observations should be made upon arrival, as well as precautions for safety. It is imperative that the assessor explain, in clear detail and multiple reiterations, how the owner needs to contain the dog, using what equipment, and exactly where the owner should have the dog upon arrival, including but not limited to:

- ❑ Where, exactly the owner should have the dog upon arrival (Indoors? In a room? Crate? Backyard? etc.).

- ❑ On what equipment (leash, collar, muzzle, etc.) the owner should have the dog upon arrival.

- ❑ How exactly the owner should be holding the equipment (e.g., the handle of the leash looped around the owner's wrist, etc.).

I much prefer to arrive safely and without the dog present if there is any possibility of the dog being aggressive toward strangers. I will then meet the owners, often hear the dog barking in the distance/some other room, time how long it takes for the dog to calm and settle, and then, finally, when I have enough behavior history and am properly prepared, conduct the Stranger test. I want to supervise the owner during the set-up of the test, double leash/double collar the dog for the assessment, to ensure the safety of all involved. I instruct the owners/fosters to not try to distract, train or influence the dog in any way during the assessment. I will always let them know that, if at any time they are uncomfortable with something I am doing, they can tell me so and we will stop the assessment. I will tell them exactly what is going to happen during the assessment, as well as behaviors I am looking for. During this preface, while I am at the same time becoming more familiar with and to the dog, I can have my assistant leave, put on a hooded sweatshirt or don a cap/hat, and have them appear as the stranger during an actual assessment. In almost all cases, I prefer to conduct a Stranger test toward the end of the consult/assessment, as it gives the dog the most time to get comfortable with me and to potentially consider me part of the territory or resources worth guarding.

The Stranger tests (and Cage Presentation tests) look at the dog's responses to unfamiliar people/strangers, and to unfamiliar people while the dog remains behind a barrier (including a leash). The behaviors we're looking to ferret out are how the dog might ultimately respond in the home when guests come, or when the dog is being walked on leash in a quiet setting and a stranger appears and approaches, or how the dog might respond while in the car and a gas station attendant approaches, etc.

In the private behavior setting, getting a read on the extent of the dog's actual problem can be difficult using just history-taking, since an owner with a problem dog often puts the dog away in another room or in a crate when guests come, or we, as trainers, immediately set the dog up for success, and manage the situation, thereby never viewing the full extent of the dog's potential. It can be useful to know what the dog is capable of doing to a stranger if and when the owners slip up in their training and management program. Some dogs get better with behavior modification and training, and others need management for life. If, as a trainer, you're coming in on the middle of an owner's training program, and they have already been working with and managing the dog, then the benefit of testing the dog may not outweigh the risk of the possible setback that testing may cause. You will have to weigh and decide whether or not the evaluation itself can add some knowledge that eclipses the setback it will inevitably cause.

Stranger testing considerations

The procedures for Stranger testing are the same as in AAP (see Chapter 6), but can be done indoors or outdoors, or both, depending on any particular behavior history from the dog.

Age factors

Until a dog reaches maturity, at about 3 to 4 years of age, its fearful and/or aggressive responses to strangers are still progressing and developing. At maturity, they usually level off, unless there is some unusually traumatic event. Therefore, responses seen here in dogs less than 1 year old are more worrisome than the same responses seen in mature dogs, since these young dogs still have potential to get worse.

Dogs that have issues with strangers will need considerably more management, attention to behavior/body language and attention to the environment than dogs without issues with strangers. These include dogs that "don't like/are afraid of men," or are generally suspicious of strangers. More successful placements include owners without the distraction or time-consumption of children. Even homes with older children can be problematic for dogs with stranger issues as pre-teens and teens are often home alone with the dog without adult supervision, and are less likely to perform any management of stranger-encounters. Teenagers' friends are often dressed in more intimidating fashion: heavy makeup, multiple piercings, and can be more varied and therefore more intimidating or frightening than regular adult strangers.

Placing dogs with issues with strangers requires finding a Level Three person or professional trainer with prior experience in managing this type of dog for the placement to be successful. Management for a dog with stranger problems is almost always a lifetime endeavor.

Using the Resource Guarding tests in the home

Whether or not to implement the AAP procedures for testing for resource guarding during an in-home behavior consultation is a bigger question than for some of the other tests. This is because we are testing using such familiar and everyday events, such as feeding the dog and giving him a bone to chew—but the predictive behaviors do not necessarily correlate one to one to those exact every day events—however, anyone bearing witness to these specific tests cannot help but be hesitant the next time they reach for that dog's bone if they witnessed him full-out snarling and lunging—but that may never have been where the dog's low threshold was going to manifest itself. That dog's low threshold during his pig's ear test may have been predicting that the dog would guard the family car, or his crate, or his owner from an approaching stranger, but now that we saw how he responded to his pig's ear test, the next person to go near him while he is chewing something will inevitably behave hesitantly, differently, and likely get a different response than usual.

Deciding when to do the Resource Guarding test

As a trainer, during a consult with an owned dog, I will test for resource guarding if:

- ❑ The dog is new to the home and there are questionable behaviors seen in the dog.
- ❑ The dog is new to the home and there are children or frail adults with the dog.
- ❑ The dog has exhibited guarding responses in certain situations.

As a trainer, during a consult with an owned dog, I will NOT test for resource guarding if:

- ❑ The dog is established in the home (has lived with the owner(s) for three or more months) and there is no history of food bowl, chew toy, or nonedible toy guarding.
- ❑ The dog is established in the home and the people are committed to the dog and would not consider re-homing or not keeping the dog.
- ❑ There are no presenting aggression issues.
- ❑ There are resource guarding issues presenting but they are mild and behavior modification work has already begun.

Procedures for testing for Resource Guarding in the home:

1. Tether the dog securely on a short leash/cable.

2. Always use an Assess-A-Hand.

3. Exclude children from observing or participating.

4. You as the trainer/behaviorist should be holding the Assess-A-Hand and performing the tests, but the owner(s) should be close by and obviously out of reach of the tether.

5. Follow the AAP procedures from Chapter 5 exactly.

Assessing a dog's reaction to children in the home

The tests associated with children in AAP can be used for a pet dog in the home or a fostered dog to see how he responds to babies and toddlers. This is especially critical when the owners or future potential owners are newly pregnant, or are planning on having or adopting a child. It may also be appropriate to include testing for response to children (or cats) whenever a dog is being considered for *any* placement, since you never know if the dog you are placing will get passed along from his original home into a home with children. It is also useful to assess a dog for new owners seeking an assessment of their recently adopted dog.

While it takes a special dog to be able to live successfully in a family with young children (less than 8 years old), many dogs that are unsuitable for homes with children can be safely placed into and live successfully in homes *without* resident and/or frequently visiting young children. Dog owners who have frequent visitation by young children should be treated the same as households with resident children, since intermittent exposure to children and less vigilant supervision can lead to an aggressive event.

The unthinkable can happen

While dogs that kill infants are extremely rare, when it does occur it is a hideous and catastrophic event. But if all it took for a dog to kill an infant was to be left alone in a room with an infant, I believe there would be many more dead infants. Not every dog is just waiting for the opportunity to be left alone in a room with an unattended infant so that he can attack. However, although rare, there are dogs with such temperaments that are unsafe and dangerous, and would, if given that opportunity, kill an infant. I have not had the opportunity to test dogs with a history of killing infants, so I can only hypothesize. I am guessing that the type of temperament that would kill an infant if the opportunity arose is that of a dog with zero to low sociability, that is easily aroused and that would likely have low aggression thresholds in multiple areas.

Using dolls in testing

A dog's response to young children is seemingly one of the most difficult behaviors to assess, since infants and toddlers cannot be used to test dogs for obvious reasons. However, using dolls is a safe and effective alternative. While it's understandable to assume that an imitation of the real thing would never fool a dog, considering his olfactory superiority and prowess, it is simply just not the case. In my experience testing thousands of shelter dogs, I have seen that their responses to dolls are often identical, like signatures, to their previous and subsequent responses to real children. And the dogs' responses to the dolls are unrelated to the dogs' responses to toys. I have informally replaced the baby doll and mechanical cat

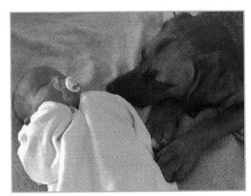

with a wadded up sweatshirt or dog toy, tested the same way and not seen the type of responses the dog has to the actual dolls. I have also taken the baby dolls and fake cats and treated them exactly as I have the toy during the toy test, and not seen the same toy behaviors.

While the information gained from using dolls is often fairly neutral and not significantly illuminating one way or the other, the real benefit of the test lies in identifying the occasional dog that falls on either end of the behavioral spectrum: those dogs that seem to adore young children, seek them out, almost prefer them to adults, and those dogs that seem to hate young children on sight; those dogs that are completely comfortable, casual and gentle while engaging with the toy cat, and those dogs that arouse immediately and lose all control around the toy cat.

Using dolls and stuffed animals in training and behavior modification programs

The baby and toddler dolls, along with the toy cat, not only make great assessment tools, but also make great training, desensitization and counter-conditioning aids while treating or helping the owner manage a problem. Baby dolls should be introduced to any parent considering or expecting a baby, and the dog should be trained how to behave while the parents nurse, change diapers, rock or give any attention to the baby. Adding actual baby smells (ointments, powders, milk, clothes from friends' real babies) and real baby sounds (tape recordings of crying, mewling babies can be purchased or homemade with the help of friends) can add to and enhance any training and behavior modification program.

Even when a dog is already living with a young child it may be valuable to test the dog with a doll. Reports from the owner about the dog's behavior history may be incomplete, unreliable or in conflict with information from other members of the household. Testing with a doll is an opportunity for you to observe the dog's reactions first hand in a controlled setting.

Dolls for testing can be found at most large chain toy stores, or toy departments in most major department stores. The best baby dolls are life-sized and life-like, and should have battery operated vocalizations and movements so they make realistic crying sounds as well as have some movement in their hands and feet.

The best toddler dolls are ones that are also life-sized, even if they're made of cloth, as long as they have large, round, realistic eyes. My Size Barbie™ and Suzy Stretch™ are two brands that work well.

Procedures for Baby and Toddler Doll testing:

The procedures for performing the Baby Doll and Toddler Doll tests are the same as in AAP (see Chapter 6), and you can choose to be the one holding the dolls and pretend to be visiting, or instruct the owners on how to hold and handle them, and have the owner(s) conduct the tests.

Make it seem real

It is important that before the dolls even appear within view of the dog that they are being handled and carried like real children, i.e. don't just grab the doll by the arm and sling it into view to begin testing.

Cat testing in the home

While the information gained from using fake cats is often fairly neutral and not significantly illuminating one way or the other, the real benefit of the test lies in identifying the occasional dog which falls on either end of the behavioral spectrum: those dogs that are completely comfortable, casual and gentle while engaging with the fake cat, and those dogs that arouse immediately and lose all control around the fake cat.

When to test

As a trainer, during a consult with an owned dog, I will perform a Cat test if /when:

- ❑ The owner is contemplating or planning on getting a cat.
- ❑ There are any reported issues with the dog and either the resident cat or a neighbor's cat.
- ❑ There is a history of killing cats.

Procedures for Cat testing:

The procedures for testing an owned dog in his home are the same as for AAP (see Chapter 6), with the following additional test if there are any reported issues with a resident cat or a neighbor's cat:

1. After double leashing/double collaring the dog (to ensure there is no chance of the dog breaking free of his equipment and doing any injury to the cat) walk the dog to within sight of the real cat.

2. Keep the dog at least 10 feet away from the real cat, and restrain him for 60 seconds.

3. After the dog has had 60 seconds to build up any frustration, cover the dog's eyes/turn his back to the action.

4. Remove the real cat and bring in the fake cat, replacing the cat at exactly the last place the dog saw the real cat.

5. Restrain the dog at a distance of 10 feet for 15 seconds and then release the dog to the fake cat.

At the writing of this book, Hasbro has made a very convincing life-like white cat that sits, meows, moves its head, purrs and has large, glowing, staring green eyes.

Dog-Dog testing in the home

When to perform the test

As a trainer, during a consult with an owned dog, I will perform a Dog-Dog test if /when:

- ❑ The dog has questionable behaviors when he sees or encounters unfamiliar or familiar dogs.
- ❑ The dog has leash reactivity issues and has an unknown history in off-leash situations with other dogs.
- ❑ The owner(s) are considering adding a second dog and there is a question about the resident dog with other dogs.

As a trainer, during a consult with an owned dog, I will NOT dog-dog test using a dog the owners are considering introducing into their home. This is not the procedure for *introducing* a new dog—this is the procedure for *testing* a dog.

For shelter and rescue personnel:

There is almost no reason I would NOT test an owned or fostered dog for dog-dog behaviors—particularly with an owner present—as it is an opportunity to see any potential resource guarding of the owner, among other issues.

Procedures for Dog-Dog testing

The procedures are exactly the same as in AAP (see Chapter 5); have the owned dog stationary and in the testing area first, and then bring in the tester-dog.

CHAPTER 8

The Trinity: Dog-Human-Environment

We have assessed the dog, but now what? While this book is all about the dog and his thresholds for aggression, equally if not more important is the human who the dog lives with and the environment in which he exists. And each point of this triangle is really equally important—identifying adoptable dogs is only one part of the trinity. There is the dog himself and his temperament and behaviors and size and instincts; there is the human or humans, with their experience, skills, time, efforts, knowledge, etc., or lack thereof; then there is the environment in which the dog and human live and move about: urban, suburban, crowded or spacious, noisy or calm, lots of visitors, scant visitors, street-walking or hiking trails, dog parks or day care, camping trips, training classes, etc., and a good dose of luck as well. In a perfect triangle, the dog gets his dream human(s) and perfect environment, the humans get their perfect pet dog, and the environment consists of all the physical attributes that contribute to harmony and success, with a great big dose of good luck to keep everyone safe and happy. But of course things are not always perfect…

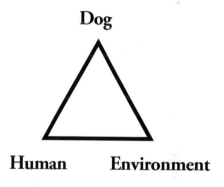

Assessing the impact of humans and the environment

In order to understand canine temperament and better assess aggression thresholds, you need to consider the humans and the environment in which the dog lives. As a trainer or a shelter worker, this may not be an easy thing for you to do but it is important to try. You can have a dog with low thresholds for aggression but, given the right human and/or right environment, that dog can be successful and lead a long, uneventful life. There are some dogs whose thresholds are so high across all categories of aggression that even with the wrong owner and/ or the wrong environment, a dog this "good" won't go "bad." Just like there are some dogs whose thresholds are so low across one or more categories of aggression that even with just the right owner and just the right environment, a dog this "bad" cannot have a successful outcome.

This triangle is important to recognize, as so often an owner will report theirs is a "good" dog, having been a successful and non-aggressive companion for years. The dog may indeed be one with high thresholds in all categories or, just as likely, the dog may have low thresholds in one or more categories, but has lived in just the right environment or with just the right person. This phenomenon is what makes the assessment so important. This can be particularly true when the owner has had the dog since he was a puppy. A puppy is small and vulnerable, and most people don't become afraid of their own dog until he is reaching adolescence—around 7 months of age. Owners of puppies with low thresholds in one or more areas usually learn to live with, dance around, and often create rituals that help thwart or stave off an aggressive event. When re-homing this dog, owners are almost never aware of any extra maneuvering they do to prevent aggression—to these owners, the dog is simply a good dog with seemingly low risk.

Another variable to consider is that today's *environment* has made it harder and harder to be a dog. There are more people. There is less open space. The economy is still not fully recovered and many people work long hours. There are more dogs, and more people with more than one dog—and therefore more dogs living with people who divide their time even further with each dog. More dogs mean more dog-dog encounters on leash and off leash, and less privacy and safe spaces for dogs. There are more reactive dogs, and hence more and more dogs gets barked at and charged at whether they are walked in an urban, suburban or rural environment, and still even more dogs become reactive because they are constantly getting charged and barked at.

Dogs are left alone more, since people are so busy. The market is flooded with toys and interactive devices with which to entertain our dogs. And while these toys and interactive devices are good things—they can provide chewing outlets, hours of activity that can help a dog actually look forward to being left alone and reduce his anxieties about it—might we also be promoting the constant, mild-to-moderate level of arousal and stimulation of our dogs? Where they used to just sleep when left alone, now they may remain in an almost constant state of arousal. More dogs attend dog day care, and interact and bond with other dogs for hours at a time. I would guess many dogs spend more time in the presence of other dogs than they do with their humans. Which again is a great thing, in the absence of any quality time between dog and human. But first choice would be the dog and human together, partnered in activities, exercise, fun, nature, play, and learning.

And despite all the good, even GREAT things that come along with reward-based dog training methods, and the improvement of dog training techniques becoming science-based and not pack- or dominance-based, the fallout has been a generation of dog trainers and humans who no longer touch, handle, *feel* a dog. We have lost the art of touch and handling. I believe that without physical touch, guidance, gentle and loving restraint, many dogs can remain in a state of constant arousal. While food is the fastest and best way to teach a dog to do anything, and is my preferred teaching tool, food *arouses*. You use food to get a keen, edgy performance. I would not want to return to the days of the choke collar and yanking the dog on his neck to get behaviors, but back then we touched and handled and communicated with our dogs via a physical connection that is simply lost today. I want to be able to take hold of my dog's collar and have her immediately understand that this is a good thing, she is safe, that when I have her by the collar she is to relax and understand I will let her know what is next.

In today's dog world we have made it so that the dog never has to do anything he does not want to do: pills are chewable and tasty, and never have to get forced down a dog's throat; we have toys for them that require no human presence to make the game fun; dogs play more with other dogs than with humans, and often have less admiration for humans—play is very powerful, and the best playmates make the best leaders and role models— perhaps than ever before.

Trainers used to be able to concentrate on just training. Most people partook of group classes as the way to give their dog basic manners and training. Now, more and more training is done privately and on an individual basis. Our training is more focused, more science-based, and much, much more humane. But trainers are faced with the job of also *inspiring* dog owners to want to do the work, and fighting against what national television, along with editing, time-constraints and entertainment, has created as a false idea of how quick and dramatic success can be.

Our human responsibility: A formula for success

Successful pet dogs come in all varieties. There are successful pet dogs with high aggression thresholds; there are also some successful pet dogs with low aggression thresholds. There are successful pet dogs with high sociability; there are successful pet dogs with low sociability. How do they do it? Is it just plain luck? Or might there be some formula for success? Some set of common features that owners of good dogs, difficult dogs and bad dogs all share? I have been studying this for the past few years in an informal way. I have amassed a list of observations common to the most successful pet owners:

Successful dog owners:

- ❑ Have their dog's attention. Attention is paramount—if your dog is looking at you, he cannot see all the things in life that can over-excite him, scare him, make him mad, etc. Successful dog owners never let eye contact go un-reinforced: they smile at their dog, say "Hi," praise him, give him a treat, tell him he is a good dog, each and every time their dog looks at them. Teach your dog to look up at you as a cue and ask for it as much as you ask for a sit. Ask for eye contact before your dog sees a squirrel, or before he sees a rabbit, or the neighbor's angry, staring dog, etc.

- ❑ Train their dogs—not just because they want them to sit when asked, but because all training (as long as it is reward-based) is communication, and the more you communicate with your dog, the more attentive and fulfilled he is. Reward-based training is fun and effective, and teaches the dog that his interactions with humans are not random. The dog can offer a behavior that can be acknowledged and reinforced, and then the human can ask for a behavior and the dog can acknowledge! This promotes more and more attention and eye contact from the dog, and better and better behaviors.

- ❑ Maintain a minimum of ten discrete behaviors they can ask for that their dogs will execute with joy. The core cues: sit, down, stay/okay, come, look at me—plus a handful of various tricks (paw, spin, sit-pretty, etc.).

- ❑ Spend quality time in nature with their dogs as often as possible. Access to nature is critical. A pet dog is an animal, first and foremost, and needs to be able to express his instincts—sniff and forage and hunt (without killing) and run and just be out in the natural environment.

- ❑ Touch and handle their dogs, confidently, gently, smoothly, proficiently, lovingly. They *feel* their dogs, find where they love to be touched and petted, find how hard or soft the dog's favorite depth of petting is, and then use touch as a reward, as a shared relaxation event, as another shared bonding event.

- ❑ Engage in partnered access to a dog's instincts. Instead of, or on top of basic manners classes, successful dog owners participate in a dog sport. There is agility, barn hunt, tracking, flyball, treibball, among many, many others. My personal favorite all-around dog sport that can fit any lifestyle and dog: Nose-work. Visit www.nacsw.net for information on the sport, classes and certified instructors. You don't have to be athletic, nor does the dog, and it inspires great teamwork and allows the dog to hunt, *with you,* for a Q-tip dipped in special essential oils, so no animals are harmed in this hunt! I recommend, in particular, the NACSW venue as it has built into its system an accommodation for all dog temperaments and abilities, and works to ensure the safety and success of dogs during the training.

- ❑ See the dog as a teammate in the sport of life. When out in public with their dogs, they are with them 100%—they don't multitask. When they take their dogs for walks, they watch their surroundings, watch their dog, they don't check texts or window shop. Successful dog owners preempt situations so that their dogs feel that the humans are in charge of the territory and will keep them safe. The most successful dog owners stay on top of their dogs and situations, see events coming before they arrive, and use training and management to thwart bad behaviors.

- ❑ Play with their own dogs more than their own dogs play with other dogs. Successful dog owners know how to play with their dogs and do so often. Their dogs admire them because they believe them to be the most fun creature—human OR dog—to be with.

- ❑ Understand that training and behavior modification are for life, and that living with a dog is hard work, filled with compromise and honoring the dog's temperament and personality.

- ❑ Share joy—in this way pet owners build a bond, forge a partnership, and earn the admiration, trust and respect of their dogs. Shared joy is play. Shared joy is a hike in nature. Shared joy is engaging in a dog sport together. Shared joy is a quiet, indoor massage. Shared joy is staying connected with dogs via conversation, eye contact, communication and by seeing the relationship as a partnership—each working to enhance the other's life.

In conclusion

"Humane society." We have lost the meaning behind the words humane society. It has become synonymous with animal shelter, but its meaning used to be a *goal*. I still believe the words should serve as a mission statement for us all. Because it is through our relationships with dogs—both in our private and public interactions—that we can model and inspire a more humane society. This comes from all sides: it is critical that shelters assess their populations carefully and make objective decisions that respect the human as much as the dog; that placement decisions are made, first and foremost, on aggression thresholds, and not on politics and statistics; that we look for not just the person's dream dog, but just as importantly, the dog's dream human and dream environment; that shelters place the needs and safety of the society as high as they place the needs of their own facility's euthanasia rates. We must always remember that dogs are not numbers, they are individual, living creatures with thresholds and traits that make or break them.

APPENDIX 1

Research on Assessing Aggression Thresholds

Research study number one

Kelley S. Bollen and Joseph Horowitz, "Behavioral evaluation and demographic information in the assessment of aggressiveness in shelter dogs." *Animal Behavioral Science,* Volume 112, July 2008

Abstract

Behavioral evaluations of 2017 shelter dogs were used for identifying dogs with aggressive tendencies and for predicting post-adoption behavior problems. Associations between failure of the behavioral evaluation and demographic factors (age, breed, and sex) and the dog's behavioral history, evaluated by logistic regression, were highly significant ($P < 0.0005$), except for "old" dogs (age > 72 months). Dogs that failed the behavior evaluation were not placed for adoption; therefore it was not possible to study prospectively the capability of behavioral evaluation to predict future aggressiveness in these dogs. Instead we developed tests for classifying dogs as aggressive or not aggressive based on their demographic factors and behavior evaluation outcomes. The results were compared retrospectively to the dogs' known behavioral histories, which were obtained at intake to the shelter. This allowed estimation of the sensitivity, specificity, and accuracy of the classification tests. The most significant postdictor (i.e., "retrospective predictor") of aggressiveness was failure of the behavioral evaluation (odds ratio 11.83, $P < 0.0005$). Among dogs that passed the behavioral evaluation, classification as "unsocial" by the behavioral evaluation was associated with nonaggressive behavior problems reported at 6-month follow-up ($P = 0.005$), and classification as "borderline" was associated with return to the shelter for aggressive behavior ($P = 0.028$). Behavioral evaluations reduced the rate of returns of adopted dogs from 19% in the year prior to their institution to 14% ($P = 0.001$) during the 2-year study period. Returns for aggression were reduced from 5% to 3.5% ($P = 0.05$), with many fewer incidents of serious aggression. The majority of dogs (86%) that failed the behavioral evaluation failed multiple component tests, indicating general aggressive tendencies in these dogs. Together with demographic information and behavioral history, behavioral evaluations can help to improve decisions regarding the disposition of shelter dogs.

Research study number two

Sara L. Bennett, et. al,"Investigating behavior assessment instruments to predict aggression in dogs." *Applied Animal Behaviour Science.* Volume 141, November 2012

Abstract

This masked controlled study evaluated a group of dogs to determine if the results of two behavior assessments detected aggression in dogs that had a history of aggression according to a validated questionnaire for measuring behavior and temperament traits in dogs. Groups of dogs with or without a history of aggression were identified from owner-completed questionnaires for 67 dogs. Any dogs that had a maximum score of no greater than 1 for any question comprising aggression factors were placed in the low/no aggression group and any dogs that had a maximum score of 2 or higher on any question comprising the aggression factors were placed in the moderate to severe aggression group. This second group was further divided to separate moderate aggression from severe aggression. Two behavior assessments, Meet Your Match (MYM)™ Safety Assessment for Evaluating Rehoming™ (SAFER™) (SAFER) and a modified version of Assess-A-Pet (mAAP), were administered to each dog in random order by assistants masked to the dogs' behavioral histories. The scores for each assessment were divided into binary categorizations (no aggression or aggression). For SAFER, the aggression category was further divided, separating dogs that showed fear, arousal or inhibited aggression from those that showed moderate aggression, and from those that showed severe aggression. The previously established categories for the mAAP of 'no issue', 'unsocial', 'borderline' and 'fail' were also used. Subtest scores for each assessment were also summed. With binary categorization, SAFER showed both lower sensitivity and specificity at 0.60 (95% confidence limits (CL) = 0.44, 0.74) and 0.50 (95% CL = 0.28, 0.72) respectively, than mAAP at 0.73 (95% CL = 0.58, 0.85) and 0.59 (95% CL = 0.36, 0.79) respectively. The odds ratio showed that an aggressive dog was 4.1-fold more likely to be classified in an aggression group by the mAAP test and 1.5 times more likely by SAFER. When the assessments were split into multiple categories, SAFER results were no longer significant, but mAAP maintained a statistically significant but weak correlation of 0.34 (P = 0.005) with historical aggression categories. SAFER testing was unable to identify dogs with moderate aggression that could potentially be addressed with behavior modification. By independently selecting acceptable levels of false positive or false negative results for the assessment, summed score results could be used in shelters as an aid to selecting dogs for adoption. Behavioral assessment results should be used in conjunction with other information such as intake history and staff observations to make an informed outcome decision for an individual dog.

APPENDIX 2

Glossary

Aligned: When the dog's eyes, head and spine are in alignment when interacting with a human or another dog.

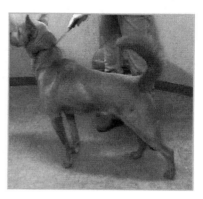

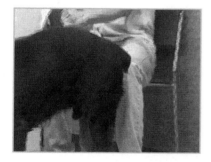

Anal swipe: When the dog's anus makes fleeting contact or brushes past an object, any part of the human, or another dog.

Anus touch: When the dog's anus makes distinct, prolonged contact with a human or object; contact lasts one second or longer. Usually seen when the dog sits on a human's shoe and ends up with his anus on top of the shoe. If the dog sits on the human's lap, sometimes the anus will plant on a different part of the human.

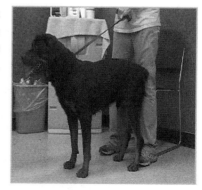

Blinking < every two seconds: When the dog blinks infrequently, less than every two seconds.

Bow: When the dog lowers his front end, elbows close to or touching the ground, while keeping his rear end up.

Chin high with throat exposed: When the dog raises, carries or holds his head in a position with his chin high and his neck arched so that his muzzle is roughly parallel with the ground, and exposes his throat.

Face diving: When the dog leaps upward at the human's face, more than once, in an intrusive, space-taking way, usually causing the human to draw back or flinch away from the dog.

Flying shoulder rub: When the dog leaps into the air with his front or all four feet and touches his shoulder to the tester.

Freeze: When the dog ceases all movement for a brief moment. Occasionally the dog will continue wagging his tail while the rest of him freezes, it is usually the tip that wags during a freeze. A freeze usually includes a tensing up of the muscles.

Freeze with head raise: When the dog ceases all body movement and raises his head higher.

Freeze with head turn: When the dog ceases all body movement and turns his head toward a human or another dog.

Front paw jab: When the dog's front paw (usually, but not always, the right paw) reaches out past the plane of the dog's nose and withdraws in a pulling motion.

Frontal body orientation: When the dog positions himself pointing his head and body directly in front of the human. Almost always occurs with alignment. Almost as precise as a perfect score for the recall-to-front position in obedience competition.

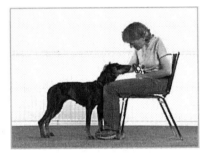

Hard eye: When the dog's eyes are open, round, with the tapetum visible. The tapetum is the reflective layer of the choroid of the eye, which gives the hard eye its characteristic marble-like, glowing quality. The brow is usually, but not always furrowed/tense.

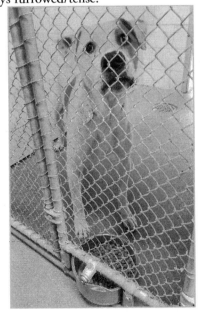 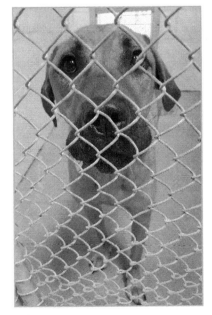

Hard stare: When the dog makes sustained eye contact lasting two seconds or longer, blinking less than every two seconds.

Head whip: When the dog moves his head abruptly and rapidly to aim at someone or something that makes contact with him.

Jump up contoured: When the dog jumps up and places his front paws on a human and makes flush or contoured physical contact; usually lasts two seconds or longer.

Jump with clasp: When the dog bends his wrists while jumping up on a human. Dog's front paws may or may not wrap around the human.

Leash bop: When the dog reaches around and pokes or nudges the leash with his nose.

Leash grab: When the dog grabs the leash into his mouth and clamps down and/or begins tugging.

Leg lift: When the dog (male or female) lifts one rear leg (or uncommonly both rear legs, usually seen in terrier type/small dogs) followed by urination or sometimes not.

Licking: Includes nose lick, sideways lick, forearm licking.

Nose lick: When the dog brings his tongue out of the front of his mouth and extends it fully over his nose. For a brief moment, the back of the dog's tongue is visible.

Sideways lick: When the tongue comes out of the front of the dog's mouth and moves from his nose down the side all the way to the back of his mouth.

Forearm licking: When the dog licks the tester's forearms so that the tongue leaves a sticky trail that can be felt by the tester minutes after the licking. Possibly done by the very back of the dog's tongue (where there is sticky saliva). Licking may occur on other parts of the tester if tester is wearing long sleeves.

Lunge away: When the dog pulls so hard on leash away from the tester as to have his front feet come off the ground or almost come off the ground.

Nose bop: When the dog's nose makes brief, poking physical contact (with no sniffing) with the human or another dog.

Penis poke: When the dog touches another dog's penis with his nose or mouth.

Poop marking: When the dog lifts one leg just prior to and sometimes during defecation, and then directs his anus high and the poop ends up falling/brushing past or landing on a high object.

Pounce off: When the dog jumps up and pushes his front paws up against a human and rebounds off. The dog is pouncing off the human. Contact is fleeting.

Rear leg hike: When the dog lifts a rear leg and steps on a human or touches the human with that leg. Any part of the dog's leg or paw may touch the human.

Shake off after contact: When the dog shakes himself off, starting with his head and shaking back from there, after any physical contact with a human.

Shoulder rub: When the dog rubs against a human or object and starts with the neck region and follows with a smear down his body.

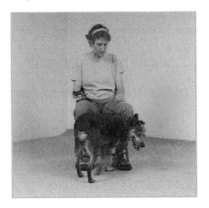 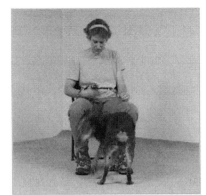

Shoulder stance: When the dog stands obliquely in front of the tester with his shoulder touching or almost touching the tester.

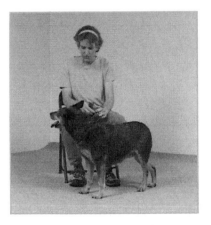

Sniffing >two seconds: When the dog sniffs something in the room or on the tester (clothes, leash, skin, rug, floor, furniture, etc.) for two seconds or longer before lifting his head up or away. If the dog sniffs an area but licks up or chews something within the two seconds, this is usually food scavenging, and not counted here.

Sociability: Two seconds or longer of gentle, physical contact made by the dog while orienting toward the human. Mounting, sniffing and biting (any teeth contact with human) are excluded.

Soft eye: When the dog squints his eyes while relaxing his brow. The dog keeps or moves his ears backward and sideways during soft eye contact. Blinking occurs more than once every two seconds during soft eye contact. The dog's lower lids come up to make the eye smaller equally to the dog's upper lids coming down to cause the squinty appearance. Commissures (corners of the mouth) are often retracted or curled up during soft eye.

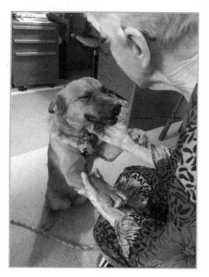 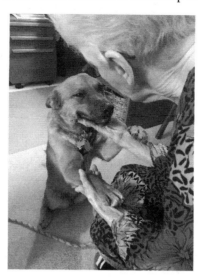

Tail carriage: Where the dog positions the base of his tail.

- ❑ Base high, tip low: This is when the base of the tail near the dog's anus is raised and the rest of the tail aims down.
- ❑ High tail carriage: A high tail carriage is when the dog's tail is above the plane of the dog's back.
- ❑ Level tail carriage: Level tail carriage is when the dog carries his tail along the same plane as the dog's back.
- ❑ Low tail carriage: A low tail carriage is when the tail is below the plane of the dog's back.
- ❑ Tucked tail: A tucked tail is when the tip is between the dog's rear legs.

Teeth clack: When the dog opens and shuts his mouth and the force of his teeth coming together makes an audible sound.

Teeth touch: When the dog's teeth (canines, incisors, pre-molars or molars) come into brief, fleeting and light physical contact with a human.

Urine mark: When the dog (male or female) urinates with a stream lasting less than five seconds. Most often preceded by sniffing.

Whale eye: When the whites of the dog's eye shows. It occurs when the dog's head moves slightly ahead of the eyeball, or when the dog moves his eyes but not his head, causing the corner to show white.

Wide panting: When the dog's mouth is parted extra wide, without having his lips retracted, while he breathes with his mouth open.

Yawn—regular: When the dog yawns.

Yawn with teeth exposed: When the dog yawns and flashes all or most of the teeth in his mouth during the widest part of the yawn.

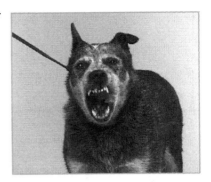

APPENDIX 3

Observations from Video Reviews of Assessments

Anus behaviors

Initially, I began to notice merely that some dogs would sit on my shoe during testing. Then I would notice that sometimes this would "gross me out" or disgust me, which I found interesting, since I am usually not in any way disgusted by dogs. I then noticed that the dogs that sat on my shoe and disgusted me would position themselves in such a way that I could feel their anus on the top of my shoes. Other dogs, with whom I was not disgusted, would position their tails or rear legs in such a way that they could sit on my shoe without their anus making contact. It had nothing to do with tail set, tail type or tail carriage. Then I began to notice that the dogs whose anuses made contact were typically the least sociable dogs, ones that commonly failed one or more parts of the full assessment. The most sociable dogs hardly ever touched their anuses to me or any other place in the testing environment. Anal glands are known for scent-marking in dogs, and it seems to me that a dog that swipes his anus all over the tester and furniture in the testing room, could, like graffiti, be tagging his signature, claiming ownership of all these things.

I was recently watching an episode of *Meerkat Manor* on Animal Planet, and was thrilled and astounded to see the first reference in any mammal, to anal marking. It was described as an "attack" and considered part of a dominance takeover by one meerkat to her injured sister. Although there was no biting or actual injury, the one meerkat repeatedly anal-swiped and shoulder rubbed all over the other meerkat.

The scent-marking cluster

I frequently see shoulder rubbing, flying shoulder rubs, shoulder stance and all the anal touching/swiping behaviors occurring together. These behaviors tend to occur in the least sociable dogs, and commonly in dogs that fail one or more portions of the test. I interpret these behaviors as a form of scent marking, and believe the dog is scent-marking or claiming the human or furniture as his own property or resource. I also see a strong correlation between these scent-marking behaviors and dogs that have low thresholds for resource guarding aggression and, maybe not as often, but also low thresholds for stranger aggression (owner/territorial guarding).

It seems to me that whether it is a human-to-human relationship or a dog-to-human relationship, the healthiest and least risky relationships are ones based significantly on respect, friendship, love, shared joy, etc., and the most risky, least healthy relationships are ones where the majority of the relationship is based on treating the other as property, or as if the other is "owned." I wonder if, when a dog shows no sociability but scent marks the tester and the furniture in the testing room throughout, he is claiming these as his own property, tagging them as resources to guard.

Most dangerous profile

I consider the large, muscular, non-sociable dog that shows many scent-marking behaviors as the most dangerous type of dog. I believe dogs that are both physically large and strong, as well as show no attachment to humans, but rub on them with their shoulders and anus, have the most potential for harm. To me, these are not in any way "pet" or "companion" dogs, but rather predators. I also believe that it is in part (along with training, relationship, bonding, bite-inhibition training) sociability that helps a dog inhibit his bite if and when the dog might otherwise choose an aggressive behavior.

Pediatric spay/neuters

As a *very new* observation, one that I am still just a spectator of, I see an abundance of what I consider scent-marking behaviors in adolescent and adult dogs suspected of, or known to have been, a pediatric spay or neuter. I define pediatric spay and neuter as sterilization performed before 6 months of age. I haven't seen enough suspected or known pediatric spay/neuters to really amass enough observations, except that I have, so far, been pretty consistently making these observations on the ones I do see.

Intense sniffing and dog-dog issues

I have noted a strong correlation between dogs that, during Sociability testing, sniff one spot for three seconds or longer and do so more than once during testing, and dogs that have low thresholds and/or any reactivity issues with other dogs. I have noticed this same sniffing during behavior consultations as well, that dogs that have issues with other dogs are most likely to come into the consultation room and intensely sniff the floors, rugs and furniture. The same holds true of the outdoor environment. These dogs will also sniff outside the consultation room, grass, trees, fence posts, etc.

It makes sense that dogs with issues with other dogs, whether they're fear-based or based in anything else, would want to gather as much information as possible about the other dogs that were in the environment before them.

Leash grabbing and resource guarding

I have noticed a correlation between dogs that grab and tug the leash during the Sociability testing and those that have low thresholds for resource guarding aggression. I'm not sure why this is, except that leaning down to pet the dog along his back is also inadvertently approaching the dog's leash, if that's indeed what he's guarding, or maybe he's guarding his body and wants to deny access to himself. The type of leash tugging most often has a very different quality to it than a fun game of tug with a pet dog. The shelter dog's tugging is more intense, jerky, violent, reckless, with more hectic chomping and re-gripping, and often includes climbing up the leash toward the tester's hands. It usually feels quite unsafe, and indeed it is unsafe, since the leash is the only point of control between dog and handler.

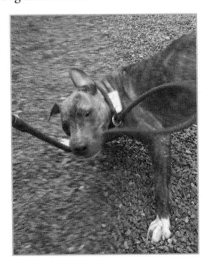 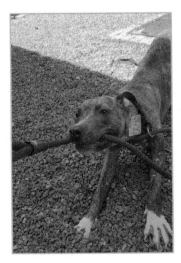

Different kinds of yawning

So far, I have observed two different kinds of yawns: one without revealing any teeth, and the other in which at some point in the event, all or most of the teeth are exposed (incisors, canines and premolars). A single dog can produce both kinds of yawns, so it does not appear to be an individual dog's style. I have observed more yawns-with-teeth-exposed in situations of competition (dog-dog, or one dog is allied with a human) or as the mildest of warnings. In my own home, I have noticed that the yawn-with-teeth occurs most often when one of my dogs is close to me and my other dog approaches—the yawn-with-teeth produced by the dog closest to me.

In conclusion

The more I assess shelter dogs, the more I videotape, the more I review the footage, the more I see. I discover new connections and behaviors all the time, even though with some familiar video clips I have viewed them hundreds of times and it feels like it is not possible to see anything more. Once I observe something new, I can then easily identify it everywhere, and then I wonder how I could possibly have ever missed it!

The benefits to breaking down behaviors into tiny, observable parts is that it takes the personal responsibility out of describing dogs. Instead of "that dog gave me a funny feeling" or "that dog scared me to death," the description becomes "the dog froze, hard-stared, blinked less than once every two seconds" or "the dog raised his tail while making frontal, aligned contact with me." These behaviors are objective, descriptive and observable by anyone, and therefore there's less room for blame and excuses.

APPENDIX 4

Recommended reading and watching to increase your knowledge of dog aggression, body language and interactions

---

Books:

Aggression in Dogs by Brenda Aloff

Aggressive Behavior in Dogs by James O'Heare

Canine Behavior, A Photo Illustrated Guide by Barbara Handelman

Canine Body Language, A Photographic Guide by Brenda Aloff

Canine Play Behavior, The Science of Dogs at Play by Mechtild Kaufer

Coaching People to Train Their Dogs by Terry Ryan

Control Unleashed by Leslie McDevitt

The Dog Vinci Code by John Rogerson

Mine! A Practical Guide to Resource Guarding by Jean Donaldson

On Talking Terms with Dogs by Turid Rugaas

Out and About With Your Dog. Dog to Dog Interactions by Sue Sternberg

Reinforcement Training for Dogs by John Fisher

The Toolbox for Building a Great Family Dog by Terry Ryan

DVDs:

Assessing Dog to Dog Interactions by Sue Sternberg

Dog-Dog Engagements Between Unfamiliar Dogs by Sue Sternberg

APPENDIX 5

Assessment Charts

This appendix contains all the charts found in Chapters 5 and 6.

Cage Presentation test responses and scoring

Note: Score A for adoptable; B for increased risk of aggression; C for high risk of aggression.

Score	Responses	Step 1	Step 2	Notes
A	Dog has low, wide, sweeping wag or circular wag at front of kennel			
A	Dog's spine is consistently curved or crescent-shaped at front of kennel			
A	Dog grovels/crawls/ approaches low to interact			
A	Dog's rear end is lower than front end at least half the time			
A	Dog carries tail level or low consistently			
A	Dog keeps eyes, head, spine unaligned during all interactions			
B	Dog's tail is carried high consistently			
B	Hackles up			
B	Dog does not approach front of kennel			
B	Dog's feet move hardly or not at all			
B	Dog's eyes, head and spine are aligned consistently while dog orients to tester			

Score	Responses	Step 1	Step 2	Notes
B	Dog barks or growls but stops within three seconds			
B	Dog consistently remains in back of kennel, whites of eyes show, stiff body			
B	Dog barks			
B	Dog growls			
B	High arousal, consistently high tail; no interaction			
C	Dog engages in repetitive behavior (leaping up and down, rebounding off kennel wall, spinning, pacing, etc.)			
C	Growling, snarling			
C	Growling with barking			
C	Dog at front of kennel lunging, barking, snapping, trying to bite			

If the dog scores mostly A responses with two or fewer B responses, in this test, proceed with Sociability testing. You will need to get the dog out of the kennel to begin Sociability testing.

Sociability test responses and scoring

Score	Responses	Step 1	Step 2	Step 3	Step 4	Notes/Observations
A	Dog has low, wide sweeping wag or circular wag					
A	Dog grovels/crawls/approaches low to interact					
A	Dog carries tail level or low consistently					
A	Dog carries tail level or just above level consistently					
A	Dog's tail is carried high but lowers during three strokes and 20 Seconds of Affection					
B	Dog's tail is high/remains high, or raises higher than plane of dog's back during interaction					
B	Three or more leash bops or nose bops					
B	Two or more jump with clasps					
B	Two or more pounce offs					
B	More than three shoulder swipes/or two shoulder stances					
B	Two or more anal swipe/anal plants					
B	Face diving (two or more)					

Score	Responses	Step 1	Step 2	Step 3	Step 4	Notes/ Observations
B	Head whip					
B	Dog puts mouth on tester					
C	Dog turns to look directly at tester—direct eye contact, blinking less than once every two seconds					
C	More than three lunge-aways					
C	Dog's feet move hardly or not at all					
C	Dog's eyes, head and spine are aligned consistently while dog orients to tester					
C	Mounts					
C	High arousal, consistently high tail					
C	Dog begins high-energy barking					
C	Dog air snaps, clacks teeth while jumping					
C	Dog puts mouth on tester, bears down, pressure					
C	Freeze/stiffening/ muscling up					
C	Dog growls					
C	Dog snaps/ attempts to bite/ bites					

Resource Guarding Toy test responses and scoring

Note: All responses are to be considered more risky with sociability scores of 5 or less.

Note: Score A for adoptable; B for increased risk of aggression; C for high risk of aggression.

Score	Responses	Step 1	Step 2	Notes/Comments
A	Dog ignores toy and offers sociability			
A	Dog ignores toy			
A	Dog appears unfamiliar with toys/won't approach or engage, or backs away from toy			
A	Dog engages toy with low arousal/interest			
A	Dog engages toy with low or medium arousal, loses interest within five seconds			
A	Dog engages toy but disengages when tester approaches			
A	Dog looks from toy to tester and back to toy again			
A	Dog shows whites of eyes/whale eye (no freezing or pausing or stiffening)			
A	Dog increases speed and intensity as test progresses			
A	Shoulder block			
B	Dog's tail raises higher over back			
B	Dog snatches resource and turns back on tester or pulls hard to a different location			

Score	Responses	Step 1	Step 2	Notes/Comments
B	Dog drops toy or leaves toy and pounces with front paws hard against tester, rebounds off tester when tester faces or approaches toy			
B	Dog hovers or briefly freezes, less than one second			
C	Dog hovers or freezes, one second or longer			
C	Dog freezes/stiffens			
C	Dog snarls			
C	Dog growls			
C	Dog snaps			
C	Dog bites Assess-A-Hand			
C	Dog ignores Assess-A-Hand and tries to bite (or successfully bites) tester			

Pig's Ear test responses and scoring

Note: All responses are considered more risky with sociability scores of 5 or less.

Note: Score A for adoptable; B for increased risk of aggression; C for high risk of aggression.

Score	Responses	Steps 1-4	Step 5-6	Notes/Comments
A	Dog chews item and begins wide wagging when tester approaches			
A	Dog shows mild/moderate interest in chewing; wags hard or harder when tester makes contact			
A	Dog shows mild/moderate interest in chewing; disengages briefly to look at tester while wagging			
A	Dog is playful with resource—tosses it in air, and/or takes resource closer to tester to chew			
A	Dog chews item and never increases in speed or intensity throughout the test			
A	Dog engages but disengages when tester approaches and offers sociability in a position not blocking access to resource			
A	Dog looks from resource to tester and back to resource again			

Score	Responses	Steps 1-4	Step 5-6	Notes/Comments
A	Dog shows whites of eyes/whale eye			
A	Dog shows more interest in the resource after the tester either steps toward or engages in testing			
A	Shoulder block			
A	Dog increases speed and intensity as test progresses/tester gets closer			
B	Dog's tail raises higher over back			
B	Dog snatches resource and turns back on tester or pulls hard to a different location			
B	Dog rubs shoulder on toy			
B	Dog drops toy or leaves pigs ear and pounces with front paws hard against tester, rebounds off tester when tester faces or approaches pigs ear			
B	Dog hovers or briefly freezes, less than one second			
C	Dog hovers or freezes one second or longer			
C	Dog freezes/stiffens			

Score	Responses	Steps 1-4	Step 5-6	Notes/Comments
C	Dog snarls			
C	Dog growls			
C	Dog snaps			
C	Dog bites Assess-A-Hand			
C	Dog skirts around Assess-A-Hand and tries to bite (or successfully bites) tester			

Food Bowl test responses and scoring

Note: All responses are considered more risky with sociability scores of 5 or less.

Note: Score A for adoptable; B for increased risk of aggression; C for high risk of aggression.

Score	Responses	Step 1	Step 2	Step 3	Step 4	Step 5	Notes
A	Dog wide wags while eating when tester touches or approaches						
A	Dog eats food at same rate during entire test						
A	Dog wide wags and looks up, ears go back, eyes squint, forehead relaxes and then goes back to eating						
A	Dog wide wags harder during back strokes and head pats						
A	Dog moves muzzle closer to tester's side of bowl when tester approaches/ touches						
A	Dog looks from food bowl to tester and back to food bowl again						

Score	Responses	Step 1	Step 2	Step 3	Step 4	Step 5	Notes
A	Dog shows whites of eyes/whale eye						
A	Dog increases speed and intensity as test progresses						
A	Shoulder block						
B	Dog's tail raises higher over back						
B	Dog hovers or briefly freezes, less than one second						
B	Dog hovers or freezes one second or longer						
B	Dog freezes/ stiffens						
C	Dog snarls						
C	Dog growls						
C	Dog snaps						
C	Dog bites Assess-A-Hand						
C	Dog skirts around Assess-A-Hand and tries to bites (or successfully bites) tester						

Dog-Dog test responses and scoring

Note: All responses are considered more risky with sociability scores of 5 or less.

Note: Score A for adoptable; B for increased risk of aggression; C for high risk of aggression.

Score	Responses	Step 1	Step 2	Step 3	Step 4	Notes
A	Dog looks away from other dog and makes sociable eye contact with tester more than once					
A	Dog changes position: shifts, turns from other dog to other points in room or toward tester multiple times					
A	Dog's ears shift positions multiple times in each procedure					
A	Dog spends over 50% of time looking at people or things other than the dog					
A	Base of dog's tail moves many times during each procedure—up, down, level, low, wide wag, no wag, wags a little					
A	Dog's eyes, head and spine are unaligned most of the time					
A	Dog's body weight is underneath him for most of the interactions—neither forward nor back					
A	Dog shifts from standing, to turning, to sitting, to bowing, to lying down multiple times					

Score	Responses	Step 1	Step 2	Step 3	Step 4	Notes
B	Dog shoulder swipes handler					
B	Dog looks at/orients toward/stares at other dog for more than 50% of the time					
B	Dog's tail raises higher over back					
B	Dog's tail remains high for most of procedures					
B	Dog raises wide hackles along back					
B	Dog raises a thin line of hackles between shoulders or along back of neck					
B	Dog mounts					
B	Dog remains still and doesn't move feet for many seconds at a time while staring at other dog					
B	Dog's eyes, head and spine are aligned more than 50% of the time					
B/C	Dog begins to whine and/or tremble					
B/C	Dog's arousal levels (breathing rate, rate of panting, excitability, etc.) rise steadily throughout test					
B/C	Dog freezes/stiffens					
B/C	Dog snarls					
B/C	Dog growls					

Score	Responses	Step 1	Step 2	Step 3	Step 4	Notes
B/C	Dog snaps					
B/C	Dog is pulling forward, or straining hard on leash toward the other dog more than 50% of the time					
B/C	Dog spends more than 50% of the time on his hind legs					
C	Dog makes hard physical contact, crashes into the other dog and/or pummels him with no communication					
C	Dog head whips (extreme handler risk)					
C	Dog tries to bite other dog					
C	Dog whips head and tries to bite handler					

Stuffed Dog test responses and scoring

Note: Score A for adoptable; B for increased risk of aggression; C for high risk of aggression.

Score	Responses	Step 1	Step 2	Step 3	Notes
B	Dog looks at/orients toward/stares at other dog for more than 50% of the time				
B	Dog's tail raises higher over back				
B	Dog's tail remains high for most of procedures				
B	Dog stiffens/freezes				
C	Dog's arousal level (breathing rate, rate of panting, excitability, etc.) rises steadily or spikes				
C	Dog whines and/or trembles				
C	Dog rushes over to stuffed dog and circles and/or sniffs				
C	Dog mounts, with or without hackles raised				
C	Dog rushes over to stuffed dog and bites/knocks down without sniffing or stopping first				
C	Dog bites stuffed dog				
C	Dog bites and shakes stuffed dog				
C	Dog bites and yanks stuffed dog to ground				
C	Dog whips head and tries to bite handler				
C	Dog resource guards/growls over, clasps, etc. stuffed dog				

Teeth Exam responses and scoring

Note: All responses are considered more risky with sociability scores of 5 or less.

Note: Score A for adoptable; B for increased risk of aggression; C for high risk of aggression.

Score	Responses	Notes
A	Dog's eyes, head and spine are not aligned, and his body is freely moving	
A	Dog wags tail level, or low and wide	
A	Dog's rear end is wagging along with tail	
A	Dog starts with a medium-high tail, but lowers during all repetitions	
A	Dog licks or nuzzles	
A	Dog remains close to tester or moves closer in between repetitions	
A	Dog may paw once or twice, or twist away but accepts all ten attempts, resisting less than 50% of the time	
A	Dog gets progressively more and more excited	
B	Dog re-orients frontally with eyes, head and spine aligned	
B	Dog's arousal level spikes	
B	Dog doesn't move his feet during most of the test and never wags tail or tail is consistently high	
B	Dog uses mouth on tester, even if with no pressure	
B	Dog jumps up and at tester, rebounds off tester's body	

Score	Responses	Notes
B	Dog's tail is high or raises during exams	
B	Dog makes direct eye contact with tester	
B	Dog head-whips toward tester	
B	Dog head-whips and mouths tester	
C	Dog gets stiff/freezes or remains stiff	
C	Dog growls	
C	Dog snarls	
C	Dog snaps	
C	Dog bites or attempts to bite	

Baby Doll testing responses and scoring

Note: All responses are considered more risky with sociability scores of 5 or less.

Note: Score A for adoptable; B for increased risk of aggression; C for high risk of aggression.

Score	Responses	Step 1	Step 2	Notes
A	Dog orients toward doll, tail low or level with sweeping or circular wag; head, eyes and spine not aligned			
A	Dog interacts with doll with non-frontal, non-aligned orientation			
A	Dog's eyes are soft and squinty; dog blinks more than once every two seconds			
A	Dog licks or nuzzles doll's fingers or hand gently			
A	Dog is respectful of doll's physical space, tail level or just higher than level (but lower than tail carriage at other environmental arousal)			
A	Dog is indifferent to doll, neither approaches to investigate nor backs off			
B	Dog backs off or avoids doll			
B	Dog steps on doll or engages with rough body contact			
B	Dog approaches doll with frontal body orientation and eyes, head and spine aligned; high tail			
B	Dog's tail remains high, eyes are open wide and hard			

Score	Responses	Step 1	Step 2	Notes
B	Dog raises hackles, either razor thin line between shoulders or full along back			
C	Dog barks at doll			
C	Dog growls at doll			
C	Dog mounts or shoulder swipes doll			
C	Dog arouses suddenly and intensely while orienting toward doll			
C	Dog leaps repeatedly at doll, highly aroused			
C	Dog grabs at doll and shakes			
C	Dog bites at doll			
C	Dog grabs doll by back of neck or head, or grabs the stomach with incisor teeth and picks up doll			

Toddler Doll responses and scoring

Note: All responses are considered more risky with sociability scores of 5 or less.

Note: Score A for adoptable; B for increased risk of aggression; C for high risk of aggression.

Score	Responses	Notes
A	Dog orients toward doll, tail low or level with sweeping or circular wag; head, eyes and spine not aligned	
A	Dog interacts with doll with non-frontal, non-aligned orientation	
A	Dog's eyes are soft and squinty; dog blinks more than once every two seconds	
A	Dog licks or nuzzles doll's fingers or hand gently	
A	Dog is respectful of doll's physical space, tail level or just higher than level (but lower than tail carriage at other environmental arousal)	
A	Dog is indifferent to doll, neither approaches to investigate nor backs off	
B	Dog backs off or avoids doll	
B	Dog steps on doll or engages with rough body contact	
B	Dog approaches doll with frontal body orientation and eyes, head and spine aligned, high tail	
B	Dog's tail remains high, dog's eyes are open and wide and hard	

Score	Responses	Notes
B	Dog barks at doll	
B	Dog growls at doll	
B	Dog raises hackles, either razor thin line between shoulders or full along back	
C	Dog mounts or shoulder swipes doll	
C	Dog arouses suddenly and intensely while orienting toward doll	
C	Dog leaps repeatedly at doll, highly aroused	
C	Dog grabs at doll and shakes	
C	Dog bites or bites at doll	
C	Dog grabs toddler doll by back of neck, hair or head	

Cat test responses and scoring

Note: All responses are considered more risky with sociability scores of 5 or less.

Note: Score A for adoptable; B for increased risk of aggression; C for high risk of aggression.

Scores	Responses	Step 1	Step 2	Notes
A	Dog looks at cat, then disengages on his own to look at tester more than twice while on leash; no tension on leash			
A	Dog sniffs air/cat briefly and disengages from cat within three seconds; no tension on leash			
A	Dog looks at cat, perks up/forward, but relaxes back or disengages within three seconds of visual contact			
A	Dog maintains low level of arousal during entire Cat Test			
A	Dog is uninterested			
A	Dog backs off or avoids cat			
B	Dog bows or barks more than once			
B	Dog bows and/or pokes at cat more than once when he is given access to cat			
B	Dog freezes while staring at cat			

Scores	Responses	Step 1	Step 2	Notes
B	Dog orients toward cat with frontal body orientation and eyes, head and spine aligned, and lowers head/ stalks			
B	Dog fixates immediately on cat, with or without trembling or whining, no disconnect within five seconds			
B	Dog arouses suddenly and intensely while orienting toward cat			
C	Dog leaps/lunges repeatedly at cat, highly aroused			
C	Dog grabs at cat and shakes, and you have to buy a new cat			

Stranger test responses and scoring

Note: All responses are considered more risky with sociability scores of 5 or less.

Note: Score A for adoptable; B for increased risk of aggression; C for high risk of aggression.

Score	Responses	SA Test	SL Test	Notes
A	Dog wags low and wide, body moves with wagging, with or without attempts to approach stranger			
A	Dog's eyes are squinty and forehead smooth; ears sideways or back			
A	Dog grovels, squints and low wags, with or without attempts to approach stranger			
A	Dog's tail is level or low			
A	Dog is bouncy, distracted, never locks onto stranger, may pounce or bow, doesn't focus on one person or object or in one direction for more than one full second			
A	Dog bows or barks more than once			
A	Dog may stare or sniff air initially, and then disengages on his own			
B	Dog stares at stranger for three full seconds before disengaging on own			

Score	Responses	SA Test	SL Test	Notes
B	Dog takes a shoulder stance, either standing or sitting during any part of the Stranger test, and watches stranger for more than three seconds			
B	Dog may growl briefly and/or back up a step or two			
B	Dog backs away; may or may not try to hide			
B	Dog arouses, pulls and strains toward stranger but scored 5 or fewer sociability points			
B	Dog doesn't move feet at all, or only one or two steps during entire test; body stiff and tense			
C	Dog erupts in barking, no recovery within five seconds			
C	Dog growls and/or snarls, no recovery within five seconds			
C	Dog stiffens, stares, no recovery within five seconds			
C	Dog remains in front of tester, frontal and aligned to stranger for more than five seconds			
C	Regardless of sociability score, dog strains, lunges, arousal spikes, high tail, no recovery within five seconds			

About the Author

Sue Sternberg has devoted her personal and professional life to helping dogs and people live together happily. Sue is known internationally for developing assessment procedures to improve the odds of successful dog adoptions based on working in shelters and as a professional dog trainer since 1981. Sue's work has greatly benefited shelters all over the world through her frequent seminars and the large number of books she has written and videos she has produced. Some of the more notable of these include *Successful Dog Adoption, Train to Adopt, Serious Fun - Play Like a Dog, Assessing Dog to Dog Interactions DVD,* and *Understanding Sociability DVD.*

After living in upstate New York much of her life, Sue recently moved to Utah, where she enjoys hiking with and competing in dog sports with her two heeler mixes, playing fiddle and scouring the desert for dinosaur fossils as an amateur paleontologist.

INDEX

A

adoptable/owned dogs, Assess-A-Pet levels, 6, 78

adopters/owners
    aggression toward owners, 86–89
    with children. *See* children
    levels of, 6, 9–10, 79–80, 86
    responsibilities, 96–97

age factors. *See* puppies

aggression thresholds, classification of, 11–12

aggression toward owners, 86–89

American Society for Prevention of Cruelty to Animals (ASPCA), 4

Asilomar Accords, 7

Assess-A-Hand, 14, 46–47

Assess-A-Pet protocol
    cage presentation, 24–27
    cat test, 68–71, 94
    development of, 1–2, 3–5
    dog-dog aggression test, 50–57, 94
    modification for private setting, 76–81
    reaction to children assessment, 63–67, 91–93
    resource guarding, 35–38, 91–92
    sociability test, 21, 27–35, 81–85
    stranger aggression test, 71–75, 90–91
    teeth exam, 58–63, 87–89
    testing overview, 13–19

Association of Professional Dog Trainers, 76

Australian Shepherds, 84

B

benefits of Assess-A-Pet, 3–4

body language of dogs
    ability to read, 79–81
    effect on adoption decisions, 4
    red flag behavior, 22–23, 83–84, 88
    scoring protocol. *See* scoring protocol
    sociability and, 22–23, 82

Boston Terriers, 84

breed rescuers, 77

breeds
    changes in shelter dog population, 8
    effect on adoption decisions, 4–5

Bulldogs, 9, 84

C

cage presentation
    overview, 16
    testing steps, 24–27

canine body language
    ability to read, 79–81
    effect on adoption decisions, 4
    red flag behavior, 22–23, 83–84, 88
    scoring protocol. *See* scoring protocol
    sociability and, 22–23, 82

cat test, 68–71, 94

Chihuahuas, 8

children
    adoptable dog levels and, 6, 10
    aggression thresholds and, 11
    assessing reaction to, 14, 63–67, 91–93
    sociability test, 32

Chows, 4

Chronicle of the Dog, The (Association of Professional Dog Trainers), 76

communication between dogs and owners, 86–89

competition training, 85

Corgis, 84

D

dog sports, 85, 97

dog-dog aggression
    defined, 12
    modification for private setting, 94
    overview, 18
    testing steps, 50–57

dogs, Assess-A-Pet levels, 78

doll testing, 14, 63–67, 91–92

E

equipment for testing, 13–14

F

food bowl test, 46–50

H

hesitant communication, 18, 36

high-crime-area shelters, 7–8, 27

I

information gathering, 78

L

leash handling tips, 27, 37, 51
live release rates, 7–8

M

management, 95–96
multiple owners, 81

O

owned/adoptable dogs, Assess-A-Pet levels, 6, 78
owners/adopters
    aggression toward owners, 86–89
    with children. *See* children
    levels of, 6, 9–10, 79–80, 86
    responsibilities, 96–97

P

physical punishment, 81
physical touch
    aggression thresholds and, 11, 96–97
    sociability test, 28, 32
    teeth exam, 58–63
pig's ear test, 40–46
play, 97
Pugs, 84
puppies
    Assess-A-Pet testing and, 15, 28–29
    sociability and, 9
    stranger aggression test and, 71, 75, 91

R

red flag behavior, 22–23, 83–84, 88. *See also* scoring
    protocol
regional influences on sociability, 8–9
resource guarding
    defined, 12
    modification for private setting, 91–92
    overview, 17–18
    testing steps, 35–38
Rottweilers, 84

S

safety
    dog-dog aggression, 18, 55
    number of testers, 13–14
    of public and families, 8, 15, 87, 89, 98
    resource guarding test, 37, 42, 50
    sociability test, 30–31, 82
    stranger test, 72, 90–91

teeth exam, 59
scoring protocol
    cage presentation, 25–26
    cat test, 70–71
    dog-dog aggression test, 52–54, 56
    overview, 20–21
    in private setting, 82
    reaction to children assessment, 64–67
    resource guarding, 38–39, 43–46, 48–50
    sociability test, 33–35
    stranger aggression test, 73–75
    teeth exam, 61–63
separation anxiety, 3, 35–38, 86
sociability
    aggression thresholds and, 11
    canine body language and, 22–23
    effect on adoption decisions, 4
    overview, 16–17
    testing steps and scoring, 21, 27–35, 81–85
spaying and neutering campaigns, 8–9
sports for dogs, 85, 97
stranger aggression
    defined, 12
    modification for private setting, 90–91
    testing steps, 71–75

T

teeth exam
    modification for private setting, 87–89
    testing steps, 58–63
toys, 36–39

W

Whippets, 84

Also available from Dogwise Publishing

Go to www.dogwise.com for more books and ebooks.

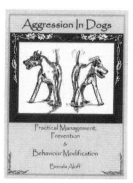

AGGRESSION IN DOGS
Practical Management, Prevention and Behaviour Modification
Brenda Aloff

Brenda Aloff's book has become the bible for identifying, understanding, and resolving aggression problems in dogs. Contains detailed training protocols to use in specific types of aggression situations and how to manage the aggressive dog for his safety and the community's. As the book says, aggression has a wide range of manifestations. And, it shows how to address reactive or aggressive behavior, with over 400 pages of text, drawings, and photographs.

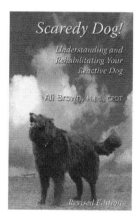

SCAREDY DOG
Understanding and Rehabilitating Your Reactive Dog
Ali Brown

When dogs growl at other dogs, lunge at people and bark at everything it's often mislabeled as "aggression." But behavior that looks like aggression is often fear-based and should be treated as such. The appropriate term for this constellation of behaviors is "reactivity." This book helps dog owners and trainers to understand the reactive dog and help him change for the better. Easy to read and understand, with photographs and graphics to help you improve behavior and solve problems.

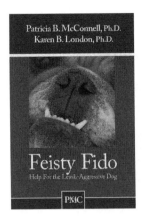

FEISTY FIDO

Help for the Leash Reactive Dog, 2nd Ed.

Patricia McConnell and Karen London

Do you have a Jekyll and Hyde dog at the other end of the leash? Is she wonderful with familiar dogs but barks and lunges at unfamiliar ones? Because of this book, thousands of people can now enjoy being out and about with their dogs instead of being anxious and nervous. Feisty Fido provides practical information about positive training ways to teach dogs how to politely walk past other dogs without causing a scene.

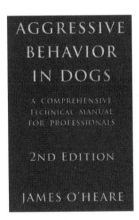

AGGRESSIVE BEHAVIOR IN DOGS

A Comprehensive Technical Manual for Professionals, 2nd Ed.

James O'Heare

A comprehensive technical manual, written for dog behavior professionals. How to assess the problem, constructing systematic behavior change programs, and case management techniques. The new second edition features a more behavioral approach to the prevention and assessment of aggression in dogs and strategies to help professionals solve aggression problems brought to them by their clients.

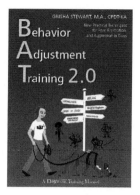

BEHAVIOR ADJUSTMENT TRAINING 2.0

Grisha Stewart, M.A., CPDT-KA

With *BAT 2.0*, trainer/author Grisha Stewart has completely overhauled Behavior Adjustment Training (BAT) to create a new efficient and practical tool for dog reactivity. *BAT 2.0* builds resilience and self-reliance by giving dogs safe opportunities to learn about people, dogs, or other "triggers." Clear enough for all readers to follow, this book also includes technical tips and bonus chapters just for dog behavior professionals. Learn how to rehabilitate aggression, frustration and fear. Grisha will teach you how to apply her technique to all dogs and puppies—and get your life back!

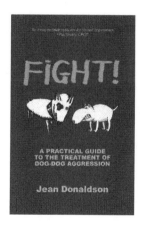

FIGHT!

A Practical Guide to the Treatment of Dog-Dog Aggression

Jean Donaldson

Fight! by Jean Donaldson is a practical guide to the treatment of dog-dog aggression. This down-to-earth manual will teach you how to use behavior modification to re-train a dog that bullies other dogs or becomes fearful when approached by other dogs.

Dogwise.com is your source for quality books, ebooks, DVDs, training tools and treats.

We've been selling to the dog fancier for more than 25 years and we carefully screen our products for quality information, safety, durability and FUN! You'll find something for every level of dog enthusiast on our website www.dogwise.com or drop by our store in Wenatchee, Washington.

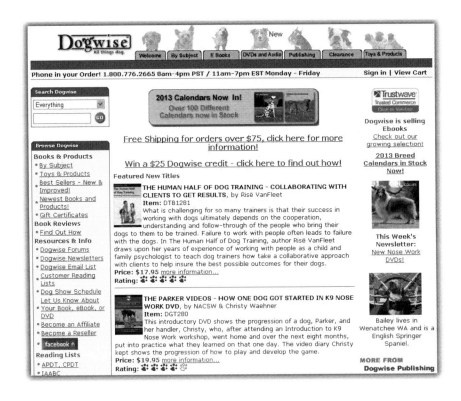

Made in the USA
San Bernardino, CA
19 January 2017